Diagnostic Testing Handbook For Clinical Decision Making

D1359012

Diagnostic Testing Handbook For Clinical Decision Making

Edited and with contributions by

Kim Goldenberg, M.D.
Associate Professor and Vice Chairman
Department of Medicine
Chief Division of General Internal Medicine
Wright State University School of Medicine
Dayton, Ohio

H. Verdain Barnes, M.D.
Professor and Chairman
Department of Medicine
Professor of Pediatrics
Wright State University School of Medicine
Dayton, Ohio

Mark M. Redding, M.D.
Resident Instructor
Department of Medicine and Pediatrics
Wright State University School of Medicine
Dayton, Ohio

Associate Editors

Steven M. Cohen, M.D.
Robert H. Edwards, M.D.
Toni I. Evans, M.D.
Elliott J. Fegelman, M.D.
Sarah A. Redding, M.D.

YEAR BOOK MEDICAL PUBLISHERS, INC.
CHICAGO • LONDON • BOCA RATON

1 2 3 4 5 6 7 8 9 0 Y 93 92 91 90 89

**Library of Congress Cataloging-in-Publication
Data**

Goldenberg, Kim.
    Diagnostic testing handbook for clinical decision
making / Kim Goldenberg, H. Verdain Barnes, Mark M.
Redding.
        p.   cm.
    Includes bibliographies and index.
    ISBN 0-8151-0487-1
    1. Function tests (Medicine)—Handbooks, manuals,
etc. 2. Diagnosis—Handbooks, manuals, etc.
I. Barnes, H. Verdain (Herman Verdain), 1935–
II. Redding, Mark M.   III. Title.
    [DNLM: 1. Diagnostic Tests, Routine—
handbooks.   QY 39 G618d]
RC71.8.G65   1989
616.075—dc19
DNLM/DLC   88-38854
for Library of Congress   CIP

Sponsoring Editor: Richard H. Lampert
Associate Managing Editor, Manuscript Services:
Deborah Thorp
Production Manager, Text and Reference/Periodicals:
Etta Worthington
Proofroom Manager: Shirley E. Taylor

To our families

Contributors

Partha Banerjee, M.D.
Clinical Professor of Medicine
Wright State University School of Medicine
Dayton, Ohio

Christopher J. Barde, M.D.
Assistant Professor of Medicine
Wright State University School of Medicine
Dayton, Ohio

H. Verdain Barnes, M.D.
Professor and Chairman
Department of Medicine
Professor of Pediatrics
Wright State University School of Medicine
Dayton, Ohio

Michael A. Baumann, M.D.
Assistant Professor of Medicine
Wright State University School of Medicine
Dayton, Ohio

Anthony W. Clarke, M.D.
Wright State University School of Medicine
Dayton, Ohio

Steven M. Cohen, M.D.
Assistant Professor of Medicine
Wright State University School of Medicine
Dayton, Ohio

Wallace M. Combs, M.D.
Wright State University School of Medicine
Dayton, Ohio

Robert H. Edwards, M.D.
Wright State University School of Medicine
Dayton, Ohio

Toni I. Evans, M.D.
Assistant Professor of Medicine
Wright State University School of Medicine
Dayton, Ohio

Curtis B. Everson, M.D.
Wright State University School of Medicine
Dayton, Ohio

Alice Faryna, M.D.
Associate Professor of Medicine
Chief, Division of Rheumatology
Wright State University School of Medicine
Dayton, Ohio

Elliott J. Fegelman, M.D.
Wright State University School of Medicine
Dayton, Ohio

Kim Goldenberg, M.D.
Associate Professor and Vice Chairman
Department of Medicine
Chief, Division of General Internal Medicine
Wright State University School of Medicine
Dayton, Ohio

Bradford H. Hawley, M.D.
Professor of Medicine and Associate Professor of Postgraduate Medicine and Continuing Education
Chief, Infectious Disease
Wright State University School of Medicine
Dayton, Ohio

Satyendra C. Gupta, M.D.
Associate Professor of Medicine
Wright State University School of Medicine
Dayton, Ohio

James V. Hennessey, M.D.
Assistant Professor of Medicine
Wright State University School of Medicine
Dayton, Ohio

Robert W. Kiefaber, M.D.
Assistant Clinical Professor of Medicine
Wright State University School of Medicine
Dayton, Ohio

Howard P. Liss, M.D.
Assistant Professor of Medicine
Wright State University School of Medicine
Dayton, Ohio

Thomas Mathews, M.D.
Associate Professor of Neurology and Pathology
Wright State University School of Medicine
Dayton, Ohio

Mark M. Redding, M.D.
*Wright State University
School of Medicine
Dayton, Ohio*

Sarah A. Redding, M.D.
*Wright State University
School of Medicine
Dayton, Ohio*

Kevin L. Riddle, M.D.
*Wright State University
School of Medicine
Dayton, Ohio*

Patricia J. Rubin, M.D.
*Wright State University
School of Medicine
Dayton, Ohio*

Mohammad G. Saklayen, M.D.
*Assistant Professor of
 Medicine
Wright State University
School of Medicine
Dayton, Ohio*

Timothy B. Sorg, M.D.
*Assistant Professor of
 Medicine
Wright State University
School of Medicine
Dayton, Ohio*

Richard D. Wetmore, M.D.
*Wright State University
School of Medicine
Dayton, Ohio*

Howard F. Wunderlich, M.D.
*Assistant Professor of
 Medicine
Wright State University
School of Medicine
Dayton, Ohio*

Preface

The ability to appropriately select and interpret diagnostic tests is a fundamental skill required in the process of clinical decision making. This book provides:

1. A clear and practical approach to the use and interpretation of diagnostic tests.
2. Easy-to-use tables that list a differential diagnosis for over 125 laboratory tests.
3. Concise and informative outlines that describe many of the laboratory findings in over 350 diseases.
4. Well-formatted tables that list test characteristics (i.e., sensitivity, specificity, and likelihood ratios) for over 140 tests.
5. A summary of diagnostic test costs, including an average and range, for over 80 diagnostic tests.

This manual was designed to provide an easy-to-use listing of diagnostic tests for medical students, house officers, and practicing physicians. Many students ask for a concise reference that focuses on diagnostic tests and that can be readily carried and used in the hospital and ambulatory setting. House officers and attending physicians often discuss the rationale for ordering as well as interpreting diagnostic tests. This text will help facilitate such discussions by consolidating much of the information that is typically available only in multiple journals and specialty textbooks, which may be difficult for busy students and physicians to access and review critically.

Tests and diseases were chosen if they were common, or associated with a potentially catastrophic outcome if the diagnosis had been missed. To keep the size and utility of the manual "user-friendly," no attempt was made to create exhaustive lists. Tests were selected and characteristics developed based on a review of the laboratory tests commonly offered by hospitals. Cut-off levels for these tests were derived primarily from the references at the end of each section. Test characteristics and cut-off levels may change based on the population studied. Footnotes are used to identify the references in which a population bias may have affected the results reported. Also, footnotes are provided when test methods were compared in the reference.

A unique strength of this manual is that its content resulted from a joint venture of 10 senior medical students at Wright State University School of Medicine and 15 of our primary care and subspecialty faculty. The students, with faculty help, reviewed several thousand articles and books using a computer-based bibliographic search and preselected criteria. This evolved from a one month student-initiated course. Our hope is that it will stimulate the reader to seek a greater depth of knowledge about laboratory testing and interpretation, and challenge the reader to keep current in this vitally important component of medical decision making.

Kim Goldenberg, M.D.
H. Verdain Barnes, M.D.
Mark M. Redding, M.D.

Acknowledgments

We wish to thank the following individuals for their contribution of time, recommendations and resources to this manual: Douglas Kaylor, Learning Resources Librarian, Fordham Health Sciences Library, Wright State University School of Medicine, Dayton, Ohio; Michael Markley, Computer Education Center, Wright State University School of Medicine, Dayton, Ohio; Kathy D. Dixon, M.D., Wright State University School of Medicine, Dayton, Ohio; Gilbert Wergowske, M.D., Assistant Professor of Medicine, Director of Ambulatory Internal Medicine, Wright State University School of Medicine, Dayton, Ohio; Corinne Jones, Computer Education Center, Wright State University School of Medicine, Dayton, Ohio; Susan Baumann, Senior Library Media Assistant, Fordham Health Sciences Library, Wright State University School of Medicine, Dayton, Ohio; June McNary, Computer Education Center, Wright State University School of Medicine, Dayton, Ohio; Helen Vafaie, Computer Education Center, Wright State University School of Medicine, Dayton, Ohio; Jinous Vafaie, Computer Education Center, Wright State University School of Medicine, Dayton, Ohio; Mazen Beetar, Computer Education Center, Wright State University School of Medicine, Dayton, Ohio; Michelle Hackett, Word Processing Consultant, Wright State University, Dayton, Ohio; Mary Faulkner, Reference/I.L.L. Librarian, Fordham Health Sciences Library, Wright State University School of Medicine, Dayton, Ohio; Kathleen Naylor, Computer Education Center, Wright State University School of Medicine, Dayton, Ohio; Aimee M. Marcellino, Computer Education Center, Wright State University School of Medicine, Dayton, Ohio; Gretchen Pfarrer, Library Assistant, Fordham

Health Sciences Library, Wright State University School of Medicine, Dayton, Ohio; and David Gillis, Library Media Assistant, Fordham Health Sciences Library, Wright State University School of Medicine, Dayton, Ohio.

Kim Goldenberg, M.D.
H. Verdain Barnes, M.D.
Mark M. Redding, M.D.

Contents

SECTION I

Selection and Interpretation of Diagnostic Tests

Kim Goldenberg, M.D.

This book has five sections dedicated to the selection and interpretation of diagnostic tests:

Section I - Selection and Interpretation of Diagnostic Tests

Section II - Tests and Associated Diseases

Section III - Diseases and Associated Tests

Section IV - Test Characteristics and Predictive Value

Section V - Cost Analysis of Selected Tests

Each section can be used, to a large extent, independent of the others, but all may be of value at some time during a patient's diagnostic evaluation. For example, in a patient who is experiencing chest pain that is atypical for myocardial infarction, a differential diagnosis of an abnormal creatine kinase may be reviewed in Section II, other abnormal diagnostic tests related to myocardial infarction in Section III, the predictive value of a creatine kinase in Section IV and the cost of a creatine kinase in different regions of the country in Section V.

This book is intended as a compendium of information for aiding the clinical decision maker in dealing with the uncertainty inherent in data gathering and the interpretation of diagnostic tests.

Section II - Tests and Associated Diseases

Test values that are minimally increased or decreased outside the normal range usually revert to a value that is within the normal range when repeated. This natural phenomenon is statistically referred to as regression toward the mean value, a value that could be determined for a person if multiple values had been obtained for a single test. Since the normal range for most tests is defined as containing 95% of the test values from a healthy population, then 2.5% of healthy persons will be above and 2.5% below the normal range. The farther the test level deviates from the normal range the less chance the value has occurred in a healthy person. Just as abnormal test values occur in healthy persons so do normal test values occur in diseased persons, depending on the stage of their disease and whether concomitant conditions that may also affect the test value are present. For example, a patient with hepatitis and dehydration may present with a normal albumin level if the effect of both conditions on serum albumin is minimal or if a decreased albumin due to hepatitis is masked by an increased albumin secondary to dehydration. **Thus, test results listed in Section II for associated diseases "may be" high or low as shown, or may be normal** in a given patient. These tables do not prioritize, preferentially select or exhaust all of the diseases which may be associated with an abnormal test but rather list those typically found in commonly used references.

Section III - Diseases and Associated Tests

The number of tests that may be abnormal in a person with a disease is often protean. When a disease is suspected or present, experts differ regarding the type and number of tests to be ordered, but they usually agree upon tests that are frequently ordered. Interpretations of these tests are generally provided in standard references for a specific disease. To succinctly review some of the tests for specific diseases, Section III is divided into subspecialty categories such as cardiology and endocrinology.

Example: for cardiogenic shock an ECG, blood tests, chest X-ray, echocardiography and a swan-ganz catheter are listed. These tests are not prioritized, preferentially selected, or exhaustive of all the tests which may be associated with a disease but rather lists those typically found in the literature. Each test listed may show: an associated description of a blood level abnormality, chronology during the disease course when the abnormality may occur, and a description of non-invasive and invasive radiologic studies or biopsies. An abnormal test described for a group of patients with the disease, however, may not be present in a particular patient because of patient variance, laboratory error, or error in diagnosis. **Thus, the test results listed in Section III for specific diseases "may be" present, absent or not necessarily ordered in a particular patient.** No attempt was made to determine which tests, for a particular disease, should be ordered for every patient suspected of having the disease. The determination of what tests are necessary and sufficient for a disease in question requires a benefit/risk and cost analysis which is outside the scope of this manual.

Section IV - Test Characteristics and Predictive Value

No test is perfect. A positive test result does not absolutely confirm a diagnosis and a negative result does not absolutely exclude a diagnosis. Knowledge of a test's sensitivity, specificity and predictive value for a disease in question can help determine the relative certainty of a disease's presence or absence based on a laboratory test(s) result.

Sensitivity or true positive is the proportion of positive tests that occur in persons with the disease. For example, the sensitivity of an acid phosphatase in patients with advanced prostate cancer (stage D) is 91%. That is, 91 out of 100 patients with prostate cancer at this stage would be expected to have a positive test result while 9 out of 100 patients would be expected to have a falsely negative result. The higher the sensitivity the more likely a negative test is to correlate with an absence of the disease in question. **Thus, one clinical use of a test with a high sensitivity is to help exclude an unlikely disease if the test result is negative.**

It should be understood when interpreting a test with a high sensitivity that the patient population used to derive the sensitivity may have had more advanced disease than the typical patient population for which the test is ordered, such as in a primary care setting. The use of a likelihood ratio may compensate, in part, for this population bias (see likelihood ratio description in this section).

4

Specificity or true negative rate is the proportion of negative tests that occur in persons without disease. For example, the specificity of an acid phosphatase in persons without prostate cancer is 92%. That is, 92 out of 100 persons without prostate cancer would be expected to have a true negative test result while 8 out of 100 persons without the disease would be expected to have a false positive result. The higher the specificity the more likely a positive test is to indicate the presence of disease. **Thus, one clinical use of a test with a high specificity is to help confirm a likely disease if the test result is positive.**

It must be considered when interpreting a test with a low specificity that the patient population used to derive the specificity may be sicker than the patient population for which the test is ordered, ie. a primary care setting. Studies do not usually indicate whether the specificity is derived from a "completely healthy" population or a population without the suspected disease, but with one or more other diseases. The use of a likelihood ratio may compensate, in part, for this population bias (see likelihood ratio description in this section).

Likelihood Ratio is the probability of a test result occurring in persons with the disease compared to the probability of a test result occurring in persons without the disease. A positive likelihood ratio may be expressed as the ratio of the true positive rate (in the diseased population) to the false positive rate (in the healthy population), or sensitivity/ (1-specificity). For example, the positive likelihood ratio of an acid phosphatase in patients suspected of having advanced prostate cancer (stage D) is 11.4, which means that a positive test is 11.4 times more likely to occur in a person with than without advanced prostate cancer. A negative likelihood ratio may be expressed as the ratio of the false negative rate (in the diseased population) to the true negative rate (in the healthy population) or (1-sensitivity)/specificity. For example, the negative likelihood ratio of an elevated acid phosphatase in patients suspected of having advanced prostate cancer is 0.1, which means that a

5

negative test is 0.1 or one-tenth as likely to occur in a person with than without prostate cancer. **Thus, one clinical use of the likelihood ratio is to conveniently combine the sensitivity and specificity into a single value.**

The likelihood ratio may, in part, negate the population biases which occur in many studies, since populations with advanced diseases may inflate the true positive rate or sensitivity (numerator) and populations without disease but with other conditions may inflate the false positive rate or one minus the specificity (denominator) resulting in little or no change in the ratio. However, this is not always predictable. For example, a 24 hour urine determination for 17-hydroxycorticosteroids has a reported sensitivity of 89% and specificity of 73% for Cushing's disease. The positive likelihood ratio is 3.3 (89%/27%). These values have been primarily reported in obese persons when the urine value was not corrected for body weight. If non-obese, as compared to obese, patients have a 26% percent decrease in sensitivity to 63% with a 26% increase in specificity to 99%, the positive likelihood ratio changes considerably to 63 (63%/1%).

The best approach, therefore, to using test characteristics such as sensitivity, specificity and likelihood ratio is to know the population from whom the test characteristics have been derived. When the population is clearly defined in the references used in this manual, we have provided that information in a footnote to the references in Section IV.

Pre-Test Probability is the probability of having a disease before any test results are known. It is primarily estimated from the history, physical examination and prevalence of the disease in the population from whom the patient comes. For example, a 70 year old male with a large, nodular prostate, bone pain and weight loss would have a high pre-test probability for having stage D, prostate cancer, e.g. 80%. Whether 80, 90 or 95% is chosen as a high probability will rarely affect the calculated outcome. For practical purposes, clinical estimates are sufficient with a 'high' probability defined as 80 to 100%, 'medium' probability = 20 to 80% and 'low' probability = 0 to 20%.

Predictive Value or post-test probability is the probability of having a disease after the test results are known. The predictive value of a test result can be determined if the pre-test probability and likelihood ratio are known. The pre-test probability is estimated on clinical grounds, as described above, and the likelihood ratio can be obtained from the tables in Section IV. These two values can be placed on the nomogram in Figure I and a predictive value obtained. For example, if the pre-test probability for the above patient example is 80% and the likelihood ratio for an acid phosphatase test is 28 in stage D prostate cancer, then the predictive value or post-test probability of disease given a positive test result (an elevated acid phosphatase) would be 99%. In contrast, if the test result is negative (a normal acid phosphatase) then the pre-test probability would still be 80%, the likelihood ratio for acid phosphatase would be 0.17, and the predictive value or post-test probability of disease given a negative test result would be 40%. Consequently, the results of this test, if positive, would help confirm the disease (99%), but if negative would not effectively exclude the disease (40%).

References to Section IV: Papers were selected using a computer-based bibliographic search system including access to Medline. Selection criteria for the articles used in this manual included papers written in English and published between January 1976 and August 1987. However if the references contained less than seven cases or the methods used for data analysis were unclear, articles dating back to 1966 and/or references from standard textbooks or reviews were used. The most recent papers were favored when the quality and number of cases were equal to or more than earlier studies. Multiple papers were often compared for consistency. Those papers in which the number of cases used to determine either the sensitivity or specificity was less than 30 are footnoted in Section IV. Footnotes are also included when the sensitivity or specificity were defined differently than in this manual.

Section V - Cost Analysis of Selected Tests

Cost is an important consideration in the clinical decision making process. Section V can assist the reader in two ways. First, it can be used to increase cost awareness, i.e., making the physician cognizant of the dollar cost of many common as well as selected specialty tests. Second, it can be used in conjunction with sensitivity, specificity and likelihood ratio data to guide one toward making diagnoses in a cost effective manner.

Test prices are listed in this section by area of the country since it is well known that health care costs often vary by region. The minimum variation from the cross-sectional average cost is 12.3%, with a maximum of 65.3% for the tests reported. Individual test prices have been listed, although many of the tests will frequently be less expensive when ordered as a panel, battery or in a provocative test as a series (i.e., growth hormone levels in an L-Dopa stimulation test, etc.). However, when ordering a typical panel of 17 to 20 tests such as selected chemistries, electrolytes and complete blood count, it should be recognized that the probability of obtaining one or more values which are outside the stated normal range is increased. Such false positives may lead to additional testing without sufficient clinical justification, thus an undesirable cost/benefit ratio. Many of the tests which are commonly referred to as "little or small ticket technology," in aggregate result in substantial cost, which in this country comprises over 50 billion dollars in health care expenditures each year.

NOMOGRAM

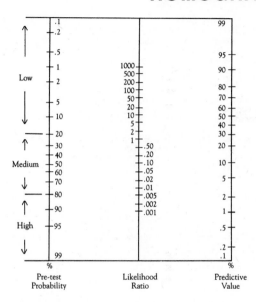

Figure 1. Nomogram for determining predictive value of a diagnostic test using the likelihood ratio. The likelihood ratios are provided in section IV. To use the nomogram, find the Pre-test Probability on the left hand scale and the Likelihood Ratio on the center scale. Draw a straight line connecting these two points and extend the line to intercept the Predictive Value on the right hand scale (modified from Fagan T.J.: *N. Engl. J. Med.* 1975;293:257. Reproduced by permission).

SECTION I REFERENCES

1. Cebul, R.D., Beck, L.H. Teaching Clinical Decision Making. New York, Praeger Publishers, 1984.

2. Galen, R.S., Gambino, S.R. Beyond Normality: The Predictive Value and Efficiency of Medical Diagnoses. New York, John Wiley and Sons, 1975.

3. Griner, P.F., Mayewski, R.J., Mushlin A.I., et al.: Selection and interpretation of diagnostic tests and procedures: Principles and applications. Ann. Intern. Med. 1981;94(2):557-600.

4. Weinstein, M.C., Fineberg, H.V. Clinical Decision Analysis. Philadelphia, W.B. Saunders, 1987.

5. Sox, H.C. Common Diagnostic Tests: Use and Interpretation. Philadelphia, American College of Physicians, 1987.

6. Griner, P.F., Panzer, R.J., Greenland, P. Clinical Diagnosis and the Laboratory: Logical Strategies for Common Medical Problems. Chicago, Year Book Medical Publishers Inc., 1986.

7. Sox, H.C., Blatt, M.A., Higgens, M.C., Marton, K.I. Medical Decision Making. Stoneham, Butterworth, 1988.

SECTION II

TESTS AND ASSOCIATED DISEASES

Robert H. Edwards, M.D.
Mark M. Redding, M.D.
Elliott J. Fegelman, M.D.
Sarah A. Redding, M.D.
Richard D. Wetmore, M.D.
Anthony W. Clarke, M.D.
Wallace M. Combs, M.D.
Curtis B. Everson, M.D.
Kevin L. Riddle, M.D.
Patricia J. Rubin, M.D.

The following data refer to blood (serum or plasma) unless indicated otherwise. These tables do not prioritize, preferentially select or exhaust all of the diseases which may be associated with an abnormal test.

11

ACID PHOSPHATASE	**RESULT MAY BE:** High Pos.	Low Neg.
Acute Renal Impairment	X	
Alcoholic Cirrhosis	X	
Benign Prostatic Hypertrophy with Infarction	X	
Bone Cancer-Metastatic	X	
Breast Cancer	X	
Bronchitis	X	
Familial Osteoectasia	X	
Gaucher's Disease	X	
Hepatitis (all types)	X	
Hyperparathyroidism	X	
Idiopathic Thrombocytopenic Purpura	X	
Lung Cancer	X	
Multiple Myeloma	X	
Niemann-Pick Disease	X	
Obstructive Jaundice	X	
Osteopetrosis	X	
Paget's Disease (advanced)	X	
Partial Translocation Trisomy 21	X	
Prostate Cancer	X	
Prostate Surgery	X	

ACTIVATED PROTHROMBIN TIME

	High Pos.	Low Neg.
Disseminated Intravascular Coagulation	X	
Factor Deficiency (I, II, V, VIII, IX, X, XI, XII)	X	
Gaucher's Disease	X	
Heparin Therapy	X	
Liver Disease, Severe	X	
Nephrotic Syndrome	X	
Vitamin K Deficiency	X	

ADRENOCORTICOTROPIC HORMONE   (ACTH)

	High Pos.	Low Neg.
Adrenogenital Syndromes	X	
Cushing's Disease due to Adrenal Hyperplasia	X	
Cushing's Disease due to Adrenal Tumor		X
Cushing's Disease due to Nodular Hyperplasia		X
Ectopic ACTH Syndrome (oat cell carcinoma of lung)	X	
Pituitary Cushing's Syndrome	X	
Primary Adrenal Insufficiency	X	
Secondary Hypoadrenalism		X

	RESULT MAY BE:	High Pos.	Low Neg.
ALBUMIN			
Alcoholic Cirrhosis			X
Burns (third degree)			X
Chronic Glomerulonephritis			X
Connective Tissue Disease			X
Cystic Fibrosis			X
Dehydration (relative increase)		X	
Exfoliative Dermatitis			X
Hepatitis (all types)			X
Hodgkin's Disease			X
Hypervitaminosis A			X
Inflammatory Bowel Disease			X
Leishmaniasis			X
Leprosy			X
Leukemia			X
Lymphomas			X
Malabsorption			X
Malnutrition			X
Multiple Myeloma			X
Nephrotic Syndrome			X
Pregnancy			X
Protein Losing Enteropathy			X
Rheumatic Fever			X
Sarcoidosis			X

ALDOLASE			
Acute Myocardial Infarction		X	
Acute Pancreatitis		X	
Acute Viral Hepatitis		X	
Burns		X	
Delirium Tremens		X	
Dermatomyositis/Polymyositis		X	
Duchenne's Muscular Dystrophy		X	
Hepatic Metastasis		X	
Hepatotoxic Drugs		X	
Intramuscular Injections		X	
Limb-Girdle Dystrophy		X	
Myotonic Dystrophy		X	
Neimann-Pick Disease		X	

RESULT MAY BE:	High Pos.	Low Neg.
(Cont.) ALDOLASE		
Prostate Cancer	X	
Rhabdomyolysis	X	
Trichinosis	X	

ALDOSTERONE

	High Pos.	Low Neg.
Adrenogenital Syndrome		X
Bartter's Syndrome	X	
Heparin Therapy		X
Pregnancy	X	
Primary Aldosteronism	X	
Pseudohyperaldosteronism	X	
Pseudohypoaldosteronism		X
Secondary Aldosteronism	X	

ALKALINE PHOSPHATASE

	High Pos.	Low Neg.
Acute Pancreatitis	X	
Alcoholic Hepatitis/Cirrhosis	X	
Amyloidosis	X	
Bile Duct Cancer	X	
Biliary Inflammation (cholecystitis)	X	
Bowel Perforation	X	
Cardiovascular Disease	X	
Childhood (normal)	X	
Chronic Active Hepatitis	X	
Chronic Heart Failure	X	
Cytomegalovirus Infection	X	
Diabetes Mellitus (uncontrolled)	X	
Drug Induced (eg: dilantin)	X	
Gallstones	X	
Healing Fracture	X	
Hepatic Abscess	X	
Hepatic Metastasis	X	
Hyperparathyroidism	X	
Hyperthyroidism	X	
Hypervitaminosis D		X
Hypophosphatasia		X
Infectious Mononucleosis	X	
Intrahepatic Cholestasis	X	

(Cont.) ALKALINE PHOSPHATASE	RESULT MAY BE: High Pos.	Low Neg.
Malnutrition		X
Obstructive Biliary Disease	X	
Osteoblastic Bone tumors (metastatic, sarcoma)	X	
Osteomalacia	X	
Paget's Disease	X	
Pancreatic Cancer	X	
Portal Cirrhosis	X	
Pregnancy	X	
Primary Biliary Cirrhosis	X	
Puberty (normal)	X	
Renal Disease	X	
Rickets	X	
Sarcoidosis	X	
Sepsis	X	
Ulcerative Colitis	X	
Viral Hepatitis	X	

ALPHA-1-ANTITRYPSIN

	High Pos.	Low Neg.
Alpha-1-Antitrypsin Deficiency		X
Cachexia		X
Cancer	X	
Emphysema		X
Hepatic Cirrhosis (infants)		X
Inflammation	X	
Lung Tissue Necrosis	X	
Malnutrition		X
Nephrosis		X
Oral Contraceptive	X	
Pregnancy	X	
Respiratory Distress (Newborns)		X

ALPHA-FETOPROTEIN

	High Pos.	Low Neg.
Anencephaly	X	
Basal Cell Cancer	X	
Breast Cancer	X	
Chronic Active Hepatitis	X	
Congenital Nephrosis	X	
Drug Induced Hepatitis	X	

(Cont.) **ALPHA-FETOPROTEIN**	**RESULT MAY BE:** High Pos.	Low Neg.
Esophageal Atresia	X	
Fallot's Tetralogy	X	
Gastric Cancer	X	
Germ Cell Tumors of the Ovary	X	
Hepatocellular Cancer	X	
Hydrocephaly	X	
Intrauterine Death	X	
Malignant Melanoma	X	
Neonatal Hepatitis	X	
Non-Seminiferous Germ Cell Testicular Tumors	X	
Pancreatic Cancer	X	
Retinoblastoma	X	
Severe Rh Isoimmunization	X	
Spina Bifida (mother's serum)	X	
Viral Hepatitis	X	
Yolk Sac Tumors	X	

AMMONIA

	High Pos.	Low Neg.
Acute Hepatic Necrosis	X	
Advanced Cirrhosis	X	
Hepatectomy	X	
Post Portacaval Anastomosis	X	
Reye's Syndrome	X	

AMYLASE

	High Pos.	Low Neg.
Acute Appendicitis	X	
Acute Pancreatitis	X	
Cerebral Trauma	X	
Cholecystitis	X	
Cirrhosis (all types)		X
Ectopic Pregnancy	X	
Hepatitis (all types)		X
Hyperlipoproteinemia Type I	X	
Intestinal Obstruction	X	
Macroamylasemia	X	
Mesenteric Thrombosis	X	
Morphine Administration	X	
Mumps	X	

(Cont.) **AMYLASE**	**RESULT MAY BE:** High Pos.	Low Neg.
Pancreatic Destruction (pancreatitis, cystic fibrosis)		X
Pancreatic Duct Obstruction (stones,tumor,stricture)	X	
Pancreatic Pseudocyst	X	
Parotitis	X	
Peptic Ulcer	X	
Post Abdominal Surgery	X	
Renal Failure (all types)	X	

ANTICENTROMERE ANTIBODIES

	High Pos.	Low Neg.
CREST Syndrome	X	
Dermatomyositis/Polymyositis	X	
Drug Induced Lupus	X	
Mixed Connective Tissue Disease	X	
Systemic Sclerosis	X	
Raynaud's Disease	X	
Sjogren's Syndrome	X	
Systemic Lupus Erythematosus	X	

ANTI-DESOXYRIBONUCLEASE-B(ANTI-DNAse-B)

	High Pos.	Low Neg.
Acute Glomerulonephritis	X	
Streptococcal Pyoderma Infection	X	

ANTI-NATIVE DNA

	High Pos.	Low Neg.
Systemic Lupus Erythematosus (Active)	X	

ANTI-NUCLEAR ANTIBODY (ANA)

	High Pos.	Low Neg.
Dermatomyositis/Polymyositis	X	
Drug-Induced Lupus	X	
Mixed Connective Tissue Disease	X	
Polymyositis	X	
Systemic Sclerosis	X	
Rheumatoid Arthritis	X	
Sjogren Syndrome	X	
Systemic Lupus Erythematosus	X	

ANTI-RIBONUCLEAR PROTEIN (ANTI-RNP)

	High Pos.	Low Neg.
Mixed Connective Tissue Disorders	X	

ANTI-SMITH ANTIBODY (Sm)	**RESULT MAY BE:**	High Pos.	Low Neg.
Systemic Lupus Erythematosus		X	

ANTI-STREPTOCOCCAL-O (ASO)

	High Pos.	Low Neg.
Pharyngitis	X	
Poststreptococcal Glomerulonephritis	X	
Rheumatic Fever	X	
Rheumatoid Arthritis	X	
Scarlet Fever	X	

ANTITHROMBIN III

	High Pos.	Low Neg.
Acute Leukemia		X
Carcinoma		X
Deep Venous Thrombosis		X
Disseminated Intravascular Coagulation		X
Familial Antithrombin III Deficiency		X
Fibrinolytic Disorders		X
Gram Negative/Gram Positive Sepsis		X
Heparin Therapy > 3 days		X
Liver Disease (chronic)		X
Myocardial Infarction	X	
Nephrotic Syndrome		X
Oral Contraceptives		X
Post-Surgery		X
Pregnancy		X
Thrombophlebitis		X
Warfarin Therapy	X	

BASOPHILS

	High Pos.	Low Neg.
Acute Phase of Infection	X	
Chickenpox	X	
Chronic Hemolytic Anemia	X	
Chronic Myelogenous Leukemia	X	
Chronic Sinusitis	X	
Hodgkin's Disease	X	
Hyperthyroidism		X
Myeloid Metaplasia	X	
Myxedema	X	
Nephrosis	X	

RESULT MAY BE:	High Pos.	Low Neg.
(Cont.) **BASOPHILS**		

	High Pos.	Low Neg.
Polycythemia Vera	X	
Post Irradiation		X
Postsplenectomy	X	
Pregnancy		X

BILIRUBIN, TOTAL

	High Pos.	Low Neg.
Biliary Obstruction (stone, tumor)	X	
Fasting	X	
Hemolysis	X	
Liver Disease (hepatitis,toxins, cirrhosis)	X	

BILIRUBIN, DIRECT

	High Pos.	Low Neg.
Biliary Obstruction (gallstone, tumor, stricture)	X	
Drug-Induced Cholestasis	X	
Dubin-Johnson Syndrome	X	
Rotor's Syndrome	X	

BILIRUBIN, INDIRECT

	High Pos.	Low Neg.
Crigler-Najjar Syndrome	X	
Gilbert's Syndrome	X	
Hemolytic Anemia	X	
Newborn Jaundice	X	

BLOOD UREA NITROGEN

	High Pos.	Low Neg.
Acromegaly		X
Acute Myocardial Infarction	X	
Drug Toxicity (eg: aminoglycosides)	X	
Gastrointestinal Bleeding	X	
Impaired Absorption (celiac disease)		X
Infancy		X
Liver Failure (hepatitis, drugs, poisoning)		X
Nephrotic Syndrome		X
Postrenal Obstruction	X	
Pregnancy		X
Prerenal Azotemia	X	
Renal Failure	X	
Starvation		X
Water Intoxication		X

RESULT MAY BE:	High Pos.	Low Neg.
c-AMP, URINE		
Familial Hypocalciuric Hypercalcemia	X	
Hypercalciuria	X	
Hyperparathyroidism (primary)	X	
Pseudohypoparathyroidism	X	
Sarcoidosis		X
Vitamin D Deficient Rickets	X	
Vitamin D Dependent Rickets	X	
Vitamin D Intoxication		X

C-PEPTIDE

	High Pos.	Low Neg.
Diabetes (Insulin Dependent)		X
Factitious Insulin Administration		X
Insulinoma	X	

C-REACTIVE PROTEIN

	High Pos.	Low Neg.
Infection	X	
Inflammation	X	
Myocardial Infarction	X	
Rheumatic Fever	X	

CALCIUM

	High Pos.	Low Neg.
Acute Renal Failure	X	
Alcoholism		X
Anticonvulsant Therapy		X
Chronic Infection	X	
Chronic Renal Failure	X	X
Cis-platinum Therapy		X
Familial Hypocalciuric Hypercalcemia	X	
Hyperparathyroidism	X	
Hyperthyroidism	X	
Hypoparathyroidism		X
Immobilization	X	
Magnesium Deficiency		X
Malabsorption		X
Malignancy	X	
Milk-Alkali Syndrome	X	
Pseudohypoparathyroidism		X
Sarcoidosis	X	

(Cont.) **CALCIUM**	**RESULT MAY BE:** High Pos.	Low Neg.
Thiazide Therapy	X	
Vitamin D Deficient		X
Vitamin D Dependent Rickets		X
Vitamin D Intoxication	X	

CALCIUM, URINE

	High Pos.	Low Neg.
Distal Renal Tubular Acidosis	X	
Drug Therapy (furosemide, mithramycin, indomethacin, phosphate, etc.)	X	
Excessive Dietary Calcium Intake	X	
Hyperparathyroidism	X	
Hyperthyroidism	X	
Idiopathic Hypercalciuria	X	
Immobilization	X	
Malignancy	X	
Paget's Disease	X	
Potassium Citrate Therapy		X
Sarcoidosis	X	
Sodium Excretion, Increased	X	
Sulfate Excretion, Increased	X	
Thiazide Diuretics		X
Vitamin D Intake, Increased	X	

CARBON DIOXIDE

	High Pos.	Low Neg.
Acetazolamide		X
Adrenal Insufficiency		X
Alcoholic Ketoacidosis		X
Bartter's Syndrome	X	
Dehydration		X
Diabetic Ketoacidosis		X
Emphysema	X	
Ethylene Glycol Ingestion		X
Lactic Acidosis		X
Metabolic Acidosis		X
Metabolic Alkalosis	X	
Methanol Ingestion		X
Paraldehyde Administration		X
Primary Aldosteronism	X	

	RESULT MAY BE:	High Pos.	Low Neg.
(Cont.) CARBON DIOXIDE			
Renal Failure			X
Respiratory Acidosis		X	
Respiratory Alkalosis			X
Salicylates			X
Severe Diarrhea			X
Severe Vomiting		X	
Starvation			X
Volume Contraction		X	

CARCINOEMBRYONIC ANTIGEN

	High Pos.	Low Neg.
Alcoholism	X	
Breast Cancer	X	
Colon Cancer	X	
Crohns Disease	X	
Emphysema	X	
Gastric Cancer	X	
Lung Cancer	X	
Pancreatic Cancer	X	
Pancreatitis	X	
Pneumonia	X	
Prostatic Cancer	X	
Smoker	X	
Transplant	X	
Ulcerative Colitis	X	

CAROTENE

	High Pos.	Low Neg.
Diabetes Mellitus (uncontrolled)	X	
Excessive Intake (carrots)	X	
High Fever		X
Hyperlipemia	X	
Hypothyroidism	X	
Liver Disease		X
Malabsorption		X

CATECHOLAMINES

	High Pos.	Low Neg.
Alcohol Intoxication	X	
Diabetic Ketoacidosis	X	
Diuretic Induced Volume depletion	X	
Ganglioblastoma	X	

RESULT MAY BE:	High Pos.	Low Neg.
(Cont.) CATECHOLAMINES		
Ganglioneuroma	X	
Hyperthyroidism	X	
Hypoglycemia	X	
Hypothyroidism	X	
Myocardial Infarction (Acute)	X	
Neuroblastoma	X	
Pheochromocytoma	X	
Post-Surgery	X	
Renal Disease	X	
Strenuous Exercise	X	

CERULOPLASMIN

	High Pos.	Low Neg.
Cancer	X	
Cirrhosis	X	
Estrogen Therapy	X	
Hyperthyroidism	X	
Infection	X	
Kwashiorkor		X
Nephrosis		X
Normal Infants		X
Oral Contraceptive	X	
Pregnancy	X	
Rheumatoid Arthritis	X	
Sprue		X
Wilson's Disease		X

CHLORIDE

	High Pos.	Low Neg.
Addisonian Crisis		X
Cystic Fibrosis (sweat test)	X	
Diabetic Ketoacidosis		X
Hyperosmolar Syndrome	X	
Hyperparathyroidism	X	
Metabolic Acidosis, Chronic	X	
Prolonged Vomiting		X
Salt-losing Nephropathy		X

RESULT MAY BE:	High Pos.	Low Neg.
CHLORIDE, URINE		
ACTH Excess	X	
Bartter's Syndrome	X	
Chronic Renal Failure		X
Diuretics	X	
Hyperchloremic Acidosis due to Chronic Renal Failure		X
Metabolic Acidosis	X	
Potassium Depletion, Severe	X	
Renal Tubular Acidosis		X
Tubulointerstitial Disease		X

CHOLESTEROL, TOTAL

	High Pos.	Low Neg.
Abetalipoproteinemia		X
Biliary Obstruction	X	
Chronic Anemia		X
Diabetes Mellitus	X	
Hyperlipoproteinemia Type IIb, III or V	X	
Hyperthyroidism		X
Hypothyroidism	X	
Liver Disease		X
Malnutrition		X
Nephrosis	X	
Pancreatic Disease	X	
Pregnancy	X	

CHOLESTEROL, HDL

	High Pos.	Low Neg.
Alcohol Intake	X	
Diabetes Mellitus		X
Estrogen Therapy	X	
Exercise	X	
Hypothyroidism		X
Increased VLDL Clearance	X	
Insulin Therapy	X	
Liver Disease		X
Nephrosis		X
Obesity		X
Progesterone Therapy		X
Serum Triglyceride Elevation		X

RESULT MAY BE:	High Pos.	Low Neg.
(Cont.) **CHOLESTEROL, HDL**		
Starvation		X
Uremia		X

COLD AGGLUTININS

Atypical Pneumonia (mycoplasmal pneumonia)	X	
Cirrhosis	X	
Parasites	X	
Viral Infections (mononucleosis, measles, mumps)	X	

COMPLEMENT C3

Gram-Negative Sepsis		X
Infectious Endocarditis		X
Partial Lipodystrophy		X
Poststreptococcal Glomerulonephritis		X
Systemic Lupus Erythematosus Nephritis		X

COMPLEMENT C4

Acute Poststreptococcal Glomerulonephritis		X
Hereditary Angioedema		X
Systemic Lupus Erythematosus Nephritis		X

COMPLEMENT CH50

Acute Phase Reactions (Acute infection, tissue injury)	X	
Hereditary Complement Deficiency		X

COOMB'S TEST, DIRECT

Autoimmune Hemolytic Anemia	X	
Erythroblastosis Fetalis	X	
Hemolytic Transfusion Reaction	X	
Drug Sensitivity	X	

COOMB'S TEST, INDIRECT

Incompatible Blood	X	
Isoimmunization (from previous transfusions)	X	

RESULT MAY BE: COPPER, SERUM	High Pos.	Low Neg.
Acute Leukemia in Remission		X
Aplastic Anemia	X	
Biliary Cirrhosis	X	
Systemic Lupus Erythematosus	X	
Hemochromatosis	X	
Hyperthyroidism	X	
Hypothyroidism	X	
Infection	X	
Iron Deficiency Anemia	X	
Kwashiorkor		X
Leukemia	X	
Malignant Lymphoma	X	
Megaloblastic Anemia of Pregnancy	X	
Nephrosis		X
Oral Contraceptive	X	
Pernicious Anemia	X	
Pernicious Anemia	X	
Rheumatoid Arthritis	X	
Wilson's Disease		X

CORTICOSTEROIDS

	High Pos.	Low Neg.
ACTH Therapy	X	
Addison's Disease		X
Adrenal Adenoma	X	
Adrenal Cancer	X	
Adrenal Hyperplasia	X	
Cushing's Disease	X	
Panhypopituitarism		X
Stress	X	

CREATINE PHOSPHOKINASE

	High Pos.	Low Neg.
Acute Myocardial Infarction	X	
Brain Infarction	X	
Cardiac Catherization with Myocardial injury	X	
Defibrillation	X	
Muscle Trauma	X	
Muscular Dystrophy	X	
Myocarditis	X	

RESULT MAY BE: (Cont.) **CREATINE PHOSPHOKINASE**	High Pos.	Low Neg.
Polymyositis/Dermatomyositis	X	
Post-Surgery	X	
Rhabdomyolysis	X	

CREATINE

High Dietary Intake of Meat	X	
Hyperthyroidism	X	
Muscle Destruction	X	
Rheumatoid Arthritis	X	
Testosterone Therapy	X	

CREATININE

Acromegaly	X	
Gigantism	X	
Ingestion of Roasted Meats	X	
Nephrotoxic Drugs	X	
Prerenal,Renal or Postrenal Obstruction	X	
Renal Failure	X	

DNA, DOUBLE STRANDED

CREST Syndrome	X	
Dermatomyositis/Polymyositis	X	
Drug induced Lupus	X	
Mixed Connective Tissue Disease	X	
Systemic Sclerosis	X	
Systemic Lupus Erythematosus	X	
Sjogren's Syndrome	X	

DNA, SINGLE STRANDED

Dermatomyositis/Polymyositis	X	
Drug Induced Lupus	X	
Hepatitis, Chronic Active	X	
Infectious Mononucleosis	X	
Mixed Connective Tissue Disease	X	
Myasthenia Gravis	X	
Systemic Sclerosis	X	
Rheumatoid Arthritis	X	

(Cont.) DNA, SINGLE STRANDED	RESULT MAY BE: High Pos.	Low Neg.
Systemic Lupus Erythematosus	X	
Sjogren's Syndrome	X	

EOSINOPHILS

Bronchial Asthma	X	
Black Widow Spider Bite	X	
Chronic Myelogenous Leukemia	X	
Dermatitis Herpetiformis	X	
Crohn's Disease	X	
Drug Allergy	X	
Echinococcus Disease	X	
Eosinophilic Gastroenteritis	X	
Erythema Multiforme	X	
Hay Fever	X	
Hodgkin's Disease	X	
Pemphigus	X	
Pernicious Anemia	X	
Phosphorus Poisoning	X	
Polyarteritis Nodosa	X	
Polycythemia Vera	X	
Post-Radiation	X	
Postsplenectomy	X	
Sarcoidosis	X	
Scarlet Fever	X	
Trichinosis	X	
Ulcerative Colitis	X	
Urticaria	X	

ERYTHROCYTE SEDIMENTATION RATE

Abcess	X	
Acute and Chronic Bacterial Infections	X	
Acute Hepatitis	X	
Carcinoma or Sarcoma	X	
Connective Tissue Diseases	X	
Hyperthyroidism	X	
Hypothyroidism	X	
Inflammatory Bowel Disease	X	
Leukemia	X	

(Cont.) **ERYTHROCYTE SEDIMENTATION RATE**	**RESULT MAY BE:** High Pos.	Low Neg.
Lymphoma	X	
Multiple Myeloma	X	
Myocardial Infarction	X	
Normal Pregnancy after Third Month	X	
Oral Contraceptives	X	
Rheumatic Fever	X	
Rheumatoid Infarction	X	
Ruptured Ectopic Pregnancy	X	
Severe Anemia	X	
Severe Renal Disease	X	
Tuberculosis	X	

ESTRADIOL

	High Pos.	Low Neg.
Amenorrhea		X
Gynecomastia	X	
Precocious Puberty in Females	X	

FECAL FAT

	High Pos.	Low Neg.
Bile Deficiency (primary biliary cirrhosis, extrahepatic bile duct obstruction)	X	
Intestinal Absorption Impairment (amyloidosis, celiac disease, tropical sprue, post-gastrectomy, lymphoma)	X	
Pancreatic Enzyme Deficiency (cystic fibrosis, pancreatic cancer, chronic pancreatitis)	X	

FERRITIN

	High Pos.	Low Neg.
Acute Liver Disease	X	
Chronic Liver Disease	X	
Hemochromatosis	X	
Hemolytic Anemia	X	
Hemosiderosis	X	
Hodgkin's Disease	X	
Hyperthyroidism	X	
Iron Deficiency Anemia		X
Leukemia	X	
Megaloblastic Anemia	X	

RESULT MAY BE:	High Pos.	Low Neg.
(Cont.) FERRITIN		
Rheumatoid Arthritis	X	
Sideroblastic Anemia	X	
Thalassemia (major/minor)	X	

FIBRIN SPLIT PRODUCTS

	High Pos.	Low Neg.
Deep Vein Thrombosis	X	
Disseminated Intravascular Coagulation	X	
Myocardial Infarction	X	
Pulmonary Embolus	X	

FIBRINOGEN

	High Pos.	Low Neg.
Abruptio Placentae		X
Acute Inflammatory Process	X	
Acute Massive Bleeding		X
Amniotic Fluid Embolism		X
Burns, Significant		X
Cardiac Surgery		X
Congenital Deficiency		X
Deep Vein Thrombosis		X
Diabetic Ketoacidosis		X
Disseminated Intravascular Coagulation		X
Eclampsia		X
Malignancy		X
Menstruation	X	
Oral Contraceptives	X	
Pregnancy	X	
Prostate Surgery		X
Sepsis (gram negative and meningococcemia)		X
Snake Bite	X	

FLUORESCENT TREPONEMAL ANTIBODY-ABSORBTION TEST (FTA-ABS)

	High Pos.	Low Neg.
Acute Genital Herpes	X	
Bejel	X	
Hypergammaglobulinemia	X	
Lupus Erythematosus	X	
Pinta	X	
Pregnancy	X	

(Cont.) FLUORESCENT TREPONEMAL ANTIBODY-ABSORBTION TEST (FTA-ABS)

	High Pos.	Low Neg.
Syphilis	X	
Yaws	X	

FOLIC ACID

	High Pos.	Low Neg.
Cancer		X
Folic Acid Therapy	X	
Hemolytic Anemia		X
Malabsorption		X
Megaloblastic Anemia		X

FOLLICLE STIMULATING HORMONE

	High Pos.	Low Neg.
Adrenal Cancer or Adenoma		X
Castration	X	
Estrogen Therapy		X
Hypophysectomy		X
Hypopituitarism		X
Klinefelter's Syndrome	X	
Menopause	X	
Oral Contraceptives		X
Ovarian Agenesis	X	
Ovarian Cancer		X
Oophorectomy	X	
Polycystic Ovarian Disease		X
Radiation, Testicle	X	
Sertoli-Cell-Only Syndrome	X	
Sheehan's Syndrome		X
Testicular Agenesis	X	
Testosterone		X
Turner's Syndrome	X	
Undescended Testicle	X	

GAMMA-GLUTAMYL TRANSPEPTIDASE (GGTP)

	High Pos.	Low Neg.
Alcoholism	X	
Childhood	X	
Cholestasis	X	
Cirrhosis	X	
Congestive Heart failure	X	

RESULT MAY BE:	High Pos.	Low Neg.
(Cont.) GAMMA-GLUTAMYL TRANSPEPTIDASE (GGTP)		
Drug Abuse (barbiturates)	X	
Fatty Liver	X	
Hepatitis	X	
Liver Metastases	X	
Obesity	X	
Obstructive Jaundice	X	
Pancreatitis	X	
Primary Biliary Cirrhosis	X	
Renal Failure	X	

GASTRIN

Antral G-Cell Hyperplasia	X	
Atrophic Gastritis	X	
Calcium Therapy	X	
Chronic Renal Failure	X	
Duodenal Ulcer	X	
Glucocorticoid Therapy	X	
Intestine Resection	X	
Pernicious Anemia	X	
Pyloric Stenosis	X	
Rheumatoid Arthritis	X	
Ulcerative Colitis	X	
Zollinger-Ellison Syndrome	X	

GLUCOSE

Acromegaly and Gigantism	X	
Acute Pancreatitis	X	
Addison's Disease		X
Chronic Pancreatitis	X	
CNS Lesions (seizure disorders, subarachnoid hemorrhage)	X	
Cushing's Disease with insulin-resistance	X	
Diabetes Mellitus	X	
Drug therapy (corticosteroids, estrogens, phenytoin, thiazides, etc.)	X	
Epinephrine Therapy	X	
Exogenous Insulin		X

RESULT MAY BE:	High Pos.	Low Neg.
(Cont.) GLUCOSE		
Extrapancreatic Tumors		X
Fructose Intolerance		X
Gastroenterostomy		X
Hypopituitarism		X
Hypothalamic Lesions		X
Hypothyroidism		X
Infant of Diabetic Mother		X
Insulinoma		X
Liver Failure (hepatitis, cirrhosis, poisoning)		X
Malnutrition		X
Oral Hypoglycemic Drugs		X
Pheochromocytoma	X	
Postgastrectomy		X
Premature Birth		X
von Gierke's Disease		X
Wernicke's Encephalopathy	X	

GROWTH HORMONE

	High Pos.	Low Neg.
Acromegaly	X	
Anorexia Nervosa	X	
Gigantism	X	

HAPTOGLOBIN

	High Pos.	Low Neg.
Most Causes of an Increased ESR	X	
Hemolysis		X
Liver Disease		X
Obstructive Liver Disease	X	

HEMOGLOBIN A1C

	High Pos.	Low Neg.
Acute Blood Loss		X
Alcoholism	X	
Chronic Renal Failure	X	
Congenital Spherocytosis		X
Diabetes Mellitus	X	
Gestational Diabetes	X	
HbS,HbC,HbD Diseases		X
Hemolytic Anemia		X

RESULT MAY BE:	High Pos.	Low Neg.
(Cont.) HEMOGLOBIN A1C		
Increased Serum Triglycerides	X	
Iron Deficiency Anemia	X	
Lead Toxicity	X	
Pregnancy		X

HEMOSIDERIN, URINE

Blood Transfusion	X	
Hemolysis	X	
Paroxysmal Nocturnal Hemoglobinuria	X	
Thalassemias	X	

HETEROPHIL ANTIBODY

Infectious Mononucleosis	X	

HISTONES

CREST Syndrome	X	
Dermatomyositis/Polymyositis	X	
Drug Induced Lupus	X	
Mixed Connective Tissue Disease	X	
Systemic Sclerosis	X	
Rheumatoid Arthritis	X	
Systemic Lupus Erythematosus	X	
Sjogren's Syndrome	X	

HLA-B27

Ankylosing Spondylitis	X	
Reiter's Syndrome	X	

HUMAN CHORIONIC GONADOTROPHIN, B SUBUNIT

Abortion	X	
Breast Cancer	X	
Choriocarcinoma	X	
Colorectal Cancer	X	
Ectopic Pregnancy	X	
Embryonal Carcinoma with Syncytiotrophoblastic Giant Cells	X	
Endometrial Cancer	X	

RESULT MAY BE:	High Pos.	Low Neg.
(Cont.) **HUMAN CHORIONIC GONADOTROPHIN, B SUBUNIT**		

	High Pos.	Low Neg.
Gastric Cancer	X	
Hematoma	X	
Hydatidiform Mole	X	
Insulinoma, Malignant	X	
Liver Cancer	X	
Malignant Melanoma	X	
Ovarian Cancer	X	
Pregnancy	X	
Seminoma with Synctiotrophoblastic Giant Cells	X	
Uterine Cervical Cancer	X	
Vulvar Cancer	X	

17-HYDROXYCORTICOSTEROIDS, SERUM AND/OR URINE

	High Pos.	Low Neg.
11-Hydroxylase Deficiency	X	
17-Hydroxylase Deficiency		X
21-Hydroxylase Deficiency		X
ACTH Deficiency		X
ACTH, Cortisone or Cortisol Therapy	X	
Addison's Disease	X	
Anorexia Nervosa		X
Cushing's Syndrome		X
Hydrocortisone or CortisoneTherapy	X	
Hyperthyroidism	X	
Hypothyroidism		X
Liver Disease, Active		X
Newborn		X
Obesity	X	
Stress -(Medical/Surgical)	X	

HYDROXYINDOLEACETIC ACID (5'HIAA), URINE

	High Pos.	Low Neg.
Carcinoid Syndrome	X	
Ingestion of Bananas, Tomatoes, Avocados, Walnuts, Eggplant, etc.	X	
Methenamine Mandelate	X	
Phenothiazine Derivatives	X	
Reserpine	X	

IRON

	RESULT MAY BE:	High Pos.	Low Neg.
Excess Destruction or Decreased Production of RBC's		X	
Hemochromatosis		X	
Hemosiderosis due to Excessive Iron Intake		X	
Iron-Deficiency Anemia			X
Liver Necrosis		X	X
Nephrosis			X
Anemia of Chronic Disease			X

IRON-BINDING CAPACITY, TOTAL

	High Pos.	Low Neg.
Acute or Chronic Bood Loss	X	
Anemia of Chronic Disease		X
Cirrhosis		X
Hemochromatosis		X
Hepatitis (all types)	X	
Iron-deficiency Anemia	X	
Nephrosis		X
Oral Contraceptives	X	X

ISOAMYLASE

	High Pos.	Low Neg.
Acute Pancreatitis	X	

JO, NUCLEAR PROTEIN ANTIGEN

	High Pos.	Low Neg.
CREST Syndrome	X	
Dermatomyositis/Polymyositis	X	
Drug Induced Lupus	X	
Mixed Connective Tissue Disease	X	
Systemic Sclerosis	X	
Systemic Lupus Erythematosus	X	
Sjogren's Syndrome	X	

17-KETOSTEROIDS,URINE

	High Pos.	Low Neg.
Adrenogenital Syndrome	X	
Hirsutism	X	
Cushing's Syndrome	X	
Masculinizing Adrenal Tumor	X	
Polycystic Ovary Disease	X	

	RESULT MAY BE:	High Pos.	Low Neg.
LACTIC ACID (LACTATE)			
Cirrhosis		X	
Exercise (strenuous)		X	
Hemorrhage		X	
Lactic Acidosis		X	
Sepsis		X	
Shock		X	

LACTIC DEHYDROGENASE

	High Pos.	Low Neg.
Acute Leukemias	X	
Acute Myocardial Infarction	X	
Burn, significant	X	
Cardiovascular Surgery	X	
Congestive Heart Failure	X	
Hemolytic Anemias	X	
Hepatitis (all types)	X	
Malignancy	X	
Pernicious Anemia, Untreated	X	
Pulmonary Embolus	X	
Nephrosis/Nephrotic Syndrome	X	
Trauma	X	
X-ray Irradiation	X	

LDH ISOENZYME I

	High Pos.	Low Neg.
Pernicious Anemia	X	

LDH ISOENZYME I AND II

	High Pos.	Low Neg.
Acute Myocardial Infarction	X	
Acute Renal Cortical Infarction	X	
Sickle Cell Crisis	X	

LDH ISOENZYME II AND III

	High Pos.	Low Neg.
Pulmonary Infarction	X	

LDH ISOENZYME III AND IV

	High Pos.	Low Neg.
Malignant Lymphoma	X	
Pulmonary Embolus with Acute Cor Pulmonale	X	
Systemic Lupus Erythematosus	X	

RESULT MAY BE:	High	Low
LDH ISOENZYME IV AND V	**Pos.**	**Neg.**
Mother Carrying Erythroblastic Fetus	X	

LDH ISOENZYME V

Dermatomyositis	X	
Early Hepatitis (all types)	X	
Electrical and Thermal Burns, Significant	X	
Prostate Cancer	X	
Trauma	X	

LEUCINE AMINOPEPTIDASE

Acute Inflammation	X	
Chronic Myelogenous Leukemia		
Hodgkin's Disease	X	X
Leukemoid Reaction	X	
Liver Disease	X	
Pregnancy	X	

LEUKOCYTES

Abscess	X	
Acute Gout	X	
Acute Hemolysis	X	
Acute Hemorrhage	X	
Acute Myocardial Infarction	X	
Aleukemic Leukemia		X
Anaphylactic Shock		X
Aplastic Anemia		X
Bacterial Infection	X	X
Brucellosis		X
Burns	X	
Cachexia		X
Cryofibrinogenemia		X
Systemic Lupus Erythematosus		X
Drugs (sulfonamides, antibiotics, analgesics, antithyroid drugs, etc.)		X
Eclampsia	X	
Epinephrine Therapy	X	
Exercise (strenuous)	X	
Felty's Syndrome		X

(Cont.) LEUKOCYTES	RESULT MAY BE: High Pos.	Low Neg.
Gangrene	X	
Gaucher's Disease		X
Hepatitis	X	X
Hypersplenism		X
Infectious Mononucleosis	X	X
Influenza	X	X
Ionizing Radiation		X
Kala-Azar		X
Malaria		X
Measles		X
Meningitis (all types)	X	
Mercury	X	
Miliary Tuberculosis		X
Multiple Myeloma		X
Myeloproliferative Diseases	X	
Paratyphoid		X
Pernicious Anemia		X
Pneumonia	X	
Psittacosis		X
Rickettsial Infections		X
Rubella		X
Septicemia	X	X
Spider Venoms	X	
Glucocorticoid Therapy	X	
Stress	X	
Tonsillitis	X	
Tularemia		X
Tumor Necrosis	X	
Typhoid		X
Uremia	X	

LIPASE

	High Pos.	Low Neg.
Acute Pancreatitis	X	
Pancreatic Duct Obstruction	X	
Perforated /Penetrating Peptic Ulcer	X	

39

LUTEINIZING HORMONE	**RESULT MAY BE:** High Pos.	Low Neg.
Anorexia Nervosa		X
Hypothyroidism		X
Polycystic Ovary Syndrome	X	
Gonad Failure/Castration	X	

LYMPHOCYTES

	High Pos.	Low Neg.
Tuberculosis	X	
Fever	X	
German Measles	X	
Hepatitis, Viral	X	
Hyperthyroidism	X	
Infectious Mononucleosis	X	
Lymphocytic Leukemia	X	
Mumps	X	
Pertussis	X	

MAGNESIUM

	High Pos.	Low Neg.
Acute Pancreatitis		X
Adrenal Insufficiency	X	
Alcoholism		X
Bowel Resection		X
Chronic Diarrhea		X
Hemodialysis	X	
Gastrointestinal Fistula		X
Hyperaldostronism		X
Hypercalcemia		X
Hyperparathyroidism	X	X
Hypoparathyroidism	X	
Idiopathic Renal Disease		X
Idiopathic Defect of Magnesium Reabsorption		X
Magnesium Poisoning	X	
Malabsorption		X
Nasogastric Suction		X
Osmotic Diuretics		X
Phosphate Deficiency		X
Protein-Calorie Malnutrition		X
Renal Disease		X
Renal Insufficiency	X	

RESULT MAY BE: MEAN CORPUSCULAR VOLUME (MCV)	High Pos.	Low Neg.
Anemia of Chronic Disease		X
Chronic alcoholism	X	
Hemolysis		X
Hyperglycemia (>600 mg/dl)	X	
Infants/Newborns	X	
Iron Deficiency Anemia		X
Leukocytosis (>50,000/cu mm)	X	
Macrocytic Anemia	X	
Methanol Poisoning	X	
Reticulocytosis (>50%)	X	
Warm Autoantibodies		X

MEAN CORPUSCULAR HEMOGLOBIN (MCH)

Hemolysis	X	
Heparin (high dose)	X	
Infants/Newborn	X	
Macrocytic Anemia	X	
Microcytic Anemias		X
Monoclonal Gammopathy	X	
Normocytic Anemia		X

METANEPHRINES, TOTAL URINE

Drugs (triamterene, benzodiazopines, hydrocortisone, chlorpromazine, etc.)	X	
Exogenous Catecholamines	X	
MAO Inhibitors	X	
Pheochromocytoma	X	

MONOCYTES

Brucellosis	X	
Chronic Ulcerative Colitis	X	
Gaucher's Disease	X	
Hodgkin's Disease	X	
Malaria	X	
Monocytic Leukemia	X	
Crohn's Disease	X	
Myeloid Metaplasia	X	
Polycythemia Vera	X	

RESULT MAY BE:	High Pos.	Low Neg.
(Cont.) **MONOCYTES**		

MONOCYTES (cont.)	High Pos.	Low Neg.
Rheumatoid Arthritis	X	
Rocky Mountain Spotted Fever	X	
Sarcoidosis	X	
Systemic Lupus Erythematosus	X	
Infective Endocarditis	X	
Tetrachlorethane Poisoning	X	
Trypanosomiasis	X	
Tuberculosis	X	
Typhus	X	

MYOGLOBIN, URINE

	High Pos.	Low Neg.
Drugs (narcotic and amphetamine toxicity, etc.)	X	
Hypothyroidism	X	
Malignant Hyperthermia	X	
Muscle Ischemia	X	
Muscle Trauma	X	
Muscular Dystrophy	X	

5' NUCLEOTIDASE

	High Pos.	Low Neg.
Bile Duct Cancer	X	
Biliary Obstruction	X	
Cholelithiasis	X	
Chronic Active Hepatitis	X	
Coronary Vascular Disease	X	
Intraheptic Cholestasis	X	
Liver Cancer (primary / secondary)	X	
Pancreatic Cancer	X	
Portal Cirrhosis	X	
Renal Failure	X	

OSMOLALITY, SERUM

	High Pos.	Low Neg.
Addison's Disease		X
Alcohol Ingestion	X	
Diabetes Mellitus/Insipidus	X	
Diuretics	X	
Ethylene Glycol Ingestion	X	
Hypercalcemia	X	
Hyponatremia		X

RESULT MAY BE:	High Pos.	Low Neg.
(Cont.) OSMOLALITY, SERUM		
Hypothyroidism		X
Mannitol Administration	X	
SIADH		X
Water Intoxication		X

PARATHYROID HORMONE

	High Pos.	Low Neg.
Chronic Renal Failure (low serum calcium)	X	
Familial Hypocalciuric Hypercalcemia (high serum calcium)	X	
Hypernephroma (high serum calcium)	X	
Lithium-Induced hypercalcemia (high serum calcium)	X	
Pregnancy (normal serum calcium)	X	
Primary Hyperparathyroidism (high serum calcium)	X	
Pseudohypoparathyroidism (low serum calcium)	X	
Hypercalcemia (other causes)		X

PHOSPHATE

	High Pos.	Low Neg.
Acromegaly	X	
Anabolic Steroids		X
Chemotherapy	X	
Diphosphate Administration	X	
Estrogen Therapy		X
Fanconi's Syndrome		X
Hyperparathyroidism	X	X
Hypoparathyroidism	X	
Idiopathic Hypercalciuria		X
Metastatic Calcification	X	
Oral Contraceptive		X
Post Renal Transplant		X
Renal Failure	X	
Renal Tubular Acidosis		X
Vitain D Dependent Rickets		X
Vitamin D Resistant Rickets		X

PHOSPHATE, URINE	RESULT MAY BE: High Pos.	Low Neg.
Acromegaly		X
Acute Renal Failure		X
Acute Tubular Necrosis, Diuretic Phase	X	
Adult-Onset Vitamin D resistant Hypophosphatemic Osteomalacia	X	
Alcoholism	X	
Chronic Renal Disease	X	
Diabetes Mellitus, (Uncontrolled)	X	
Dietary Intake, Decreased		X
Familial Hypophosphatemic Rickets	X	
Fibrous Dysplasia	X	
Glycosuria	X	
Hyperparathyroidism	X	
Hypomagnesemia	X	
Hypoparathyroidism		X
Metabolic Acidosis	X	
Metabolic Alkalosis	X	
Neurofibromatosis	X	
Renal Failure		X
Respiratory Acidosis		X
Sporadic Hypophosphatemic Osteomalacia	X	

PLATELET COUNT

	High Pos.	Low Neg.
Aplastic Anemia		X
Connective Tissue Diseases	X	X
Cytotoxic and Immunosuppressive Therapy		X
Disseminated Intravascular Coagulation		X
Drugs (thiazide diuretics, alcohol, digoxin, aspirin)		X
Folate Deficiency		X
Heparin Administration		X
Idiopathic Thrombocytopenic Purpura		X
Inflammatory Bowel Diseases	X	
Iron Deficiency	X	
Leukemia	X	
Lymphoma or Cancer	X	
Myelodysplasia		X
Myeloproliferative Syndromes	X	
Pernicous Anemia		X

RESULT MAY BE:	High Pos.	Low Neg.
(Cont.) PLATELET COUNT		
Post Blood Transfusions		X
Post Epinephrine Therapy	X	
Post Treatment with Vitamin B12	X	
Postsplenectomy	X	
Pregnancy Complication		X
Thrombotic Thrombocytopenic Purpura		X
Viral Infection		X

POTASSIUM

	High Pos.	Low Neg.
Acidosis	X	
Acute Leukemia		X
Acute Renal Diseases	X	
Addison's Disease	X	
Alcoholism		X
Alkalosis		X
Amphotericin B Therapy		X
Captopril Therapy	X	
Chronic Interstitial Nephritis		X
Extensive Tissue Injury	X	
Familial Hypokalemic Paralysis		X
Gastrointestinal (fluid losses: vomiting,diarrhea, salivary fistulas)		X
Hemolysis	X	
Hyporeninemic Hypoaldosteronism	X	
Laxative Abuse		X
Magnesium Deficiency		X
Mineralocorticoid Excess (Cushing's,Bartter's, Liddle's)		X
Nonsteroidal Anti-inflammatory Agents	X	
Poor Dietary Uptake		X
Potassium Penicillin	X	
Potassium-Sparing Diuretics	X	
Potassium Salt Substitute Use	X	
Potassium-Wasting Diuretics		X
Renal Disease		X
Renal Tubular Acidosis	X	X
Rhabdomyolysis	X	
Tumor Lysis	X	
Villous Adenoma		X

POTASSIUM, URINE	RESULT MAY BE:	High Pos.	Low Neg.
Acute Leukemia		X	
Acute Metabolic Acidosis			X
Acute Oliguric Renal Failure			X
Addison's Disease			X
Antibiotics (carbenicillin, amphotericin, etc.)		X	
Bartter's Syndrome		X	
Chronic Interstitial Nephritis			X
Chronic Metabolic Acidosis		X	
Glucocorticoid Excess		X	
Hypoaldosteronemia			X
Hyporeninemia			X
Licorice Ingestion		X	
Liddle's Syndrome		X	
Magnesium Deficiency		X	
Potassium Intake Increased		X	
Potassium Wasting Diuretics			
Renal Failure			X
Renal Tubular Acidosis		X	
Ureterosigmoidostomy		X	

PM-1, NUCLEAR ANTIGENS

	High Pos.	Low Neg.
CREST Syndrome	X	
Dermatomyositis/Polymyositis	X	
Drug Induced Lupus	X	
Mixed Connective Tissue Disease	X	
Systemic Sclerosis	X	
Systemic Lupus Erythematosus	X	
Sjogren's Syndrome	X	

PORPHOBILINOGEN, URINE

	High Pos.	Low Neg.
Lead Poisoning	X	
Metabolic Disease (erythropoietic, hepatic or erythrohepatic)	X	
Porphyria (acute intermittent, varigate and coproporphyria)	X	

	RESULT MAY BE:	High Pos.	Low Neg.
PROTEIN, TOTAL			
Decreased Albumin			X
Hodgkin's Disease			X
Inflammatory Bowel Disease			X
Leukemias			X
Macroglobulinemia		X	
Malnutrition			X
Multiple Myeloma		X	X
Sarcoidosis		X	

PROTHROMBIN TIME

	High Pos.	Low Neg.
Anticoagulant Therapy	X	
Biliary Obstruction	X	
Disseminated Intravascular Coagulation	X	
Drugs (coumadin and drugs which decrease the clearance of coumadin)	X	
Factors I,II,V,VII, or X Deficiency	X	
Fat Malabsorption	X	
Hypervitaminosis A	X	
Liver Disease, Severe	X	
Polycythemia	X	
Salicylate Intoxication	X	
Vitamin K Deficiency	X	

RENIN

	High Pos.	Low Neg.
Adrenocortical Hypertension		X
Bartter's Syndrome	X	
Chronic Renal Failure	X	
Drugs (propanolol, clonidine, reserpine, etc.)		X
Drugs (thiazides, estrogens, minoxidil, etc.)	X	
Essential Hypertension	X	X
Increased Plasma Volume		X
Last Half of Menstrual Cycle	X	
Pheochromocytoma	X	
Pregnancy (normal)	X	
Primary Aldosteronism		X
Reduced Plasma Volume	X	
Renal Hypertension	X	
Secondary Aldosteronism	X	

RETICULOCYTE COUNT	RESULT MAY BE: High Pos.	Low Neg.
Aplastic Anemia		X
Chronic Infection		X
Chronic Renal Failure	X	X
Hemolytic Anemia	X	X
Hemorrhage (acute and chronic)	X	
Hereditary Spherocytosis	X	
Iron-deficiency Anemia		X
Leukemia	X	X
Pernicious Anemia		X
Radiation Therapy		X
Sickle Cell Disease	X	X
Sideroblastic Anemia		X
Thalassemia		X

SODIUM

	High Pos.	Low Neg.
Addison's Disease		X
Cushing's Syndrome	X	
Diarrhea		X
Diuretic Therapy		X
Hyperaldosteronism	X	
Inadequate Thirst Mechanism (coma, hypothalmic disease, age)	X	
Metabolic Acidosis with Excretion of Cations and Increased Anions		X
Nephrosis		X
Polyuria	X	X
Pseudohyponatremia		X
Profuse Sweating	X	
Renal Disease	X	
Replacement of Water and Salt Loss with Free Water		X
SIADH		X

SODIUM, URINE

	High Pos.	Low Neg.
Acute Tubular Necrosis	X	
Aldosterone, Increased		X
Angiotensin II Increased		X
Bartter's Syndrome	X	
Chronic Renal Failure	X	

(Cont.) **SODIUM, URINE**	High Pos.	Low Neg.
Glucocorticoid Excess		X
Glucocorticoid Deficiency	X	
Hydronephrosis	X	
Hyponatremia		X
Interstitial Nephritis due to Analgesic Abuse	X	
Mannitol, Dextran or Glycerol Therapy	X	
Medullary Cystic Disease	X	
Milk-Alkali Syndrome	X	
Post-Obstructive Diuresis	X	
Prerenal Azotemia		X
Pyelonephritis	X	
Renin Secretion, Decreased	X	
Salt Intake, Decreased		X
Salt Intake, Increased	X	
Salt Losing Nephropathy	X	
SIADH, (Compared to Serum Sodium)	X	
Sodium Wasting Diuretics	X	
Tubulointerstitial Disease	X	

STOOL FOR OCCULT BLOOD

Colon cancer	X	
Diverticulosis	X	
Inflammatory Bowel Disease	X	
Ingested Blood	X	
Ingestion of Undercooked Meat	X	
Intestinal Polyps	X	
Ischemic Bowel Disease	X	
Peptic Ulcer Disease	X	
Vitamin C Overdose	X	

STOOL FOR WBC's

Pseudomembranous Colitis	X	
Infectious Diarrhea (*Shigella, Salmonella, E. Coli* invasive strains, *Yersinia*)	X	
Ulcerative Colitis	X	

TESTOSTERONE	**RESULT MAY BE:** High Pos.	Low Neg.
Adrenogenital Syndrome	X	
Klinefelter's Syndrome		X
Male Hypogonadism		X
Polycystic Ovary Diseases	X	

TRANSFERRIN

	High Pos.	Low Neg.
Chronic Infections		X
Hemochromatosis		X
Hemolytic Anemia		X
Iron Deficiency Anemia	X	
Iron Excess		X
Kwashiorkor		X
Malignancy		X
Nephrosis		X
Oral Contraceptives	X	
Pregnancy Late	X	
Thalassemia		X
Viral Hepatitis	X	

TRIGLYCERIDES

	High Pos.	Low Neg.
Acute Myocardial Infarction	X	
Alcoholism	X	
Congenital Abetalipoproteinemia	X	
Diabetes Mellitus	X	
Familial Hyperlipidemia	X	
Gout	X	
Hypothyroidism	X	
Malnutrition		X
Nephrotic Syndrome	X	X
Pancreatitis	X	
von Gierke's Disease	X	

T3 RIA (TRIIODOTHYRONINE)

	High Pos.	Low Neg.
Euthyroid Sick Syndrome		X
Estrogen Therapy	X	
Euthyroid Patient with Cirrhosis, Uremia or Malnutrition		X
Exogenous T4		X
Hyperthyroidism	X	

(Cont.) **T3 RIA (TRIIODOTHYRONINE)**	High Pos.	Low Neg.
Hypothyroidism		X
Oral Contraceptives	X	
Pregnancy	X	
T3 Thyrotoxicosis	X	
Thyroid Binding Globulin Deficiency		X

T3 RU (RESIN UPTAKE)

Hyperthyroidism	X	
Hypothyroidism		X
Medications (estrogens, etc.)		X
Medications (phenytoin,steroids,heparin,aspirin, etc.)	X	
Nephrotic Syndrome	X	
Oral Contraceptives		X
Pregnancy		X

T4 FREE

Amiodarone Therapy	X	
Grave's Disease	X	
Heparin Therapy	X	
Hyperemesis Gravidarum	X	
Primary Hypothyroidism		X
Propanalol	X	
Secondary Hypothyrodism		X
T3 Hyperthyroidism		X
T4 Hyperthyroidism	X	
Tertiary Hypothyroidism		X

THYROID ANTIMICROSOMAL ANTIBODY

Grave's Disease	X	
Hashimoto's Thyroiditis	X	
Juvenile Thyroiditis	X	
Nontoxic Nodular Goiter	X	
Primary Myxedema	X	
Subacute Thyroiditis	X	
Thyroid Adenoma	X	
Thyroid Cancer	X	

RESULT MAY BE: THYROID ANTI-THYROGLOBULIN ANTIBODY	High Pos.	Low Neg.
Acute Nonsuppurative Thyroiditis	X	
Grave's Disease	X	
Hashimoto's Thyroiditis	X	
Thyroid Cancer	X	
Toxic Adenoma	X	

URIC ACID

Anemia (hemolytic)	X	
Cytotoxic Drugs	X	
Diuretics	X	
Fanconi's Syndrome	X	
Gout	X	
Hypothyroidism	X	
Leukemia	X	
Parathyroid Diseases (hyper and hypo)	X	
Polycystic Kidney Disease	X	
Renal Failure	X	
Toxemia of Pregnancy	X	
Uricosuric Drugs (salycilates, probenecid, allopurinol)		X
Wilson's Disease		X

VDRL

Atypical Pneumonia	X	
Infectious Mononucleosis	X	
Leprosy	X	
Lymphogranuloma Venereum	X	
Malaria	X	
Rat-bite Fever	X	
Relapsing Fever	X	
Syphilis	X	
Systemic Lupus Erythematosus	X	
Typhus Fever	X	

VASOACTIVE INTESTINAL PEPTIDE

Ganglioneuroblastoma	X	
VIPoma	X	

VMA, URINE	**RESULT MAY BE:** High Pos.	Low Neg.
Drugs (L-dopa, maladixic acid)		X
Drugs (MAO inhibitors, methyl dopa, ethanol, clofibrate, etc)		X
Exogenous Catecholamines	X	
Foods (bananas, vanilla, coffee, etc.)		X
Neuroblastoma	X	
Pheochromocytoma	X	

VITAMIN B$_{12}$

	High Pos.	Low Neg.
Crohn's Disease		X
Diphyllobothrium Latum Infection		X
Hypothyroidism		X
Leukemia	X	
Liver Disease	X	
Malabsorption		X
Pernicious Anemia		X
Polycythemia Vera	X	
Pregnancy		X

SECTION II REFERENCES

1. Braunwald, E., et al. (ed): Harrison's Principles of Internal Medicine, 11th Ed. New York, McGraw-Hill, 1987.

2. Conn , H. F., Conn, R. B. (eds): Current Diagnosis, 6th Ed. Philadelphia, W.B. Saunders, 1980.

3. Gomella, L. G., Braen, G. R., Olding, M.: Clinician's Pocket Reference, 5th Ed. Norwalk, Appleton-Century-Croft, 1986.

4. Henry, J. B.: Clinical Diagnosis and Management of Laboratory Methods, 17th Ed. Philadelphia, W.B. Saunders, 1984.

5. Jones, H. X. Jr. and Seegar Jones, H.: Novak's Textbook of Gynecology, 10th Ed. Baltimore, Williams & Wilkins, 1981.

6. Rudolph, A. M.: Pediatrics, 18th Ed. Norwalk, Appleton-Lange, 1987.

7. Tietz, N. W. (ed): Clinical Guide to Laboratory Tests. Philadelphia, W.B. Saunders, 1983.

8. Vaughan, V. C., Behrman, R. E. (eds): Nelson Textbook of Pediatrics, 13th Ed. Philadelphia, W.B. Saunders, 1987.

9. Wallach, J. Interpretation of Diagnostic Tests: A synopsis of Laboratory Medicine, 4th Ed. Boston, Little, Brown, 1986.

10. Williams, R. H. (ed) Textbook of Endocrinology, 6th Ed. Philadelphia, W.B. Saunders, 1981.

11. Wyngaarden, J. B., Smith, L. H. Jr. (eds); Cecil Textbook of Medicine, 17th Ed. Philadelphia, W.B. Saunders, 1985.

SECTION III

Diseases and Associated Tests

Elliott J. Fegelman, M.D.
Robert H. Edwards, M.D.
Richard D. Wetmore, M.D.
Wallace M. Combs, M.D.
Kevin L. Riddle, M.D.

Mark M. Redding, M.D.
Sarah A. Redding, M.D.
Anthony W. Clarke, M.D.
Curtis B. Everson, M.D.
Patricia J. Rubin, M.D.

CARDIOLOGY — Satyendra C. Gupta, M.D.
Robert W. Kiefaber, M.D.

ENDOCRINOLOGY — James V. Hennessey, M.D.
Partha Banerjee, M.D.

GASTROENTEROLOGY — Christopher J. Barde, M.D.

HEMATOLOGY-ONCOLOGY — Michael A. Baumann, M.D.

INFECTIOUS DISEASE — Bradford H. Hawley, M.D.
Timothy B. Sorg, M.D.
Howard F. Wunderlich, M.D.

NEPHROLOGY — Mohammad G. Saklayen, M.D.

NEUROLOGY — Thomas Mathews, M.D.

PULMONARY — Howard P. Liss, M.D.

RHEUMATOLOGY — Alice Faryna, M.D.

CARDIOLOGY

The number, types and priority of tests ordered must be individualized for each patient, consequently the tests listed for each disease in this section are not prioritized and are not exhaustive.

ANGINA PECTORIS
- ECG - May be normal, show non-specific, or ischemic ST-T wave changes.
- BLOOD - Possible findings (dependent on etiology) include: elevated cholesterol and triglycerides, decreased hemoglobin and hematocrit, hypoxia or hypercapnia, increased fibrinogen, ESR elevation associated with autoimmune, vasculitis or T_4 changes (*ie*, hyper or hypothyroidism).
- STRESS TEST - With or without Thallium: Ischemic ST-T changes and ventricular dysfunction or a combination of these may be seen. Thallium scan may show reversible ischemia.
- AMBULATORY ECG (HOLTER) RECORDING - May show ischemic ST-T changes. Also useful in Prinzemetal's angina: shows marked ST elevation and/or arrythmias during chest pain.
- CARDIAC CATHETERIZATION - Helps localize and quantify coronary obstruction and assess ventricular function (*ie*, ejection fraction).
- See MYOCARDIAL INFARCTION

AORTIC DISSECTION
- ECG - May show left ventricular hypertrophy, arrhythmias or signs of pericarditis. If dissection involves the coronary ostium, it may show evidence of infarction or ischemia.
- RADIOGRAPHY

    Chest Radiograph - May show widened mediastinum and/or calcification in the aortic knob and descending aorta with a lateral shift.

    MRI/CT Scan - Will often show the site of dissection.

    Aortography - Typically shows the site of the tear (usually necessary if surgical therapy is contemplated).

ARTERIO-VENOUS FISTULA, PULMONARY
- BLOOD - Decreased a-v O_2 difference, elevated PCO_2 may be seen.
- CHEST RADIOGRAPH - May show large pulmonary artery and pulmonary vein fistula.
- SELECTIVE PULMONARY ARTERIOGRAPHY - Typically shows the extent and distribution of the fistula.

CARDIOGENIC SHOCK
- ECG - May show infarction, progressive ischemia, arrythmias and changes compatible with a ventricular aneurysm.

- •BLOOD - Lactic acidosis, hypocapnia or hypoxia and leukocytosis may be seen.
- •CHEST RADIOGRAPH - Usually cardiac enlargement or frank pulmonary edema and/or cephalad blood flow pattern.
- •ECHOCARDIOGRAM - With Doppler may show abnormal ventricular wall motion and function or valvular disease.
- •SWAN-GANZ CATHETER - May show O_2 saturation "step-up" suggesting rupture of the ventricular septum. Giant V waves may be seen with elevated pulmonary capillary wedge pressure in acute mitral regurgitation, ventricular septal defect and CHF.

CARDIOMYOPATHIES
HYPERTROPHIC
- •CHEST RADIOGRAPH - Minimal cardiomegaly with prominent left ventricle and left atrium may be seen.
- •ECG - Left ventricular hypertrophy, left atrial enlargement, abnormal Q waves (pseudoinfarction) and intraventricular conduction defects may be seen.
- •ECHOCARDIOGRAM - Increase in the thickness of the interventricular septum, systolic anterior motion (SAM) of the anterior mitral leaflet, normal or reduced left ventricular end-diastolic dimension and midsystolic closure of the aortic valve are often seen. Doppler studies show abnormal gradient across left ventricular outflow tract.
- •RADIONUCLIDE STUDIES - Left ventricular cavity may be obliterated and ventricular septum thickened.
- •CARDIAC CATHETERIZATION - Diminished left ventricular compliance (increased end-diastolic pressure), exaggerated systolic contraction, mitral regurgitation and left ventricular outflow gradient may be seen. Gradient across left ventricular outflow tract can be calculated.

DILATED
- •CHEST RADIOGRAPH - Moderate to marked cardiomegaly (predominantly left ventricular), pulmonary venous hypertension and pulmonary congestion may be seen.
- •ECG - Atrial and ventricular enlargement, and poor R wave progression in the precordial leads are frequent. Other possible findings include atrial and/or ventricular arrhythmia, intraventricular conduction defect and ST-T wave changes.

- •ECHOCARDIOGRAM - Left and right ventricle dilatation, atrial enlargement, increased ventricular end-systolic and end-diastolic volumes with decreased ejection fraction are typical. Mural thrombi may be seen.
- •RADIONUCLIDE STUDIES - Left and right ventricle dilatation, global wall motion abnormalities and decreased ejection fraction are typical. Gallium Scan may show increased uptake during subacute inflammatory stage.
- •CARDIAC CATHETERIZATION - Left ventricular dilatation with systolic dysfunction, mitral regurgitation, tricuspid regurgitation, elevated right and left filling pressures, diminished cardiac output, and filling defects due to mural thrombi are common.

RESTRICTIVE
- •CHEST RADIOGRAPH - Normal heart size or minimal cardiomegaly may be seen.
- •ECG - Low voltage, intraventricular conduction defect and/or atrioventricular conduction defect may be seen.
- •ECHOCARDIOGRAM - Symmetrical increase in left and right ventricle mass and septal thickness are typical. Small or normal left ventricular cavity may be seen. Two dimensional echocardiogram in amyloidosis may show myocardial "sparkling."
- •RADIONUCLIDE STUDIES - Small or normal left ventricle. Diffuse uptake of Technetium Pyrophosphate (TcPP) in amyloidosis.
- •CARDIAC CATHETERIZATION - Typically shows decreased left ventricular compliance, "Square root" sign in ventricular pressure tracings, increased left and right sided filling pressures, pulmonary capillary wedge pressure greater than right atrial pressure by 10 mm Hg or more. Pulmonary systolic pressure greater than 50 mm Hg may be seen.

CONGENITAL HEART DISEASE
ATRIAL SEPTAL DEFECT
- •ECG - Right axis deviation, mild right ventricular conduction delay (rSR' or rsR' in right precordial leads) and right ventricular hypertrophy may be seen, especially in ostium secundum defect.
- •ECHOCARDIOGRAM - Increase in right atrial and right ventricular dimensions and flattened or paradoxical septal motion. Doppler can estimate systemic and pulmonary blood flow and pulmonary to systemic flow ratio.

- **CHEST RADIOGRAPH** - Right atrial and ventricle enlargement, prominent pulmonary artery and branches and increased pulmonary vascular markings may be seen.
- **CARDIAC CATHETERIZATION** - Shows abnormal flow pattern, and estimates pulmonary vascular resistance, pulmonary hypertension and shunt magnitude. Oxygen saturation step-up may be seen at level of right atrium.

COARCTATION OF THE AORTA
- **ECG** - Left ventricular hypertrophy is typical.
- **ECHOCARDIOGRAM/DOPPLER**- Left ventricular hypertrophy or dilatation, and other lesions such as bicuspid aortic valve may be seen.
- **CHEST RADIOGRAPH**- Left ventricular enlargement, rib notching and/or "figure three" sign may be seen.
- **BARIUM ESOPHOGRAM** - May demonstrate E sign or reversed "3" sign.
- **CARDIAC CATHETERIZATION** - Shows the site and extent of coarctation.

PATENT DUCTUS ARTERIOSUS
- **ECG** - Left ventricular hypertrophy and left atrial enlargement may be seen.
- **CHEST RADIOGRAPH** - Left ventricular and atrial enlargement, and dilatation of the proximal pulmonary arteries may be seen. Later, dilated central pulmonary arteries with attenuated peripheral vessels and calcification of the ductus may be seen.
- **ECHOCARDIOGRAM** - Left ventricular hypertrophy and left atrial and aortic root enlargement may be seen. Two dimensional echocardiography may show ductus in short axis.

PULMONARY ATRESIA
- **ECG** - Right ventricular hypertrophy is typical.
- **ECHOCARDIOGRAM** - Complete or partial absence of the pulmonary valve is seen.
- **CHEST RADIOGRAPH** - Right ventricular enlargement is typical.

PULMONARY STENOSIS
- **ECG** - Right axis deviation, right ventricular hypertrophy and right atrial enlargement are typical.
- **ECHOCARDIOGRAM** - Shows thickened pulmonary valve leaflets with domed stenotic valve.

•CHEST RADIOGRAPH - Right ventricular hypertrophy and right atrial enlargement may be seen with severe stenosis. Post-stenotic dilatation of main and left pulmonary artery is commonly seen.

TETRALOGY OF FALLOT
•ECG - Right ventricular hypertrophy and occasional right atrial enlargement may be seen.
•BLOOD - Polycythemia and decreased O_2 saturation are usually seen late in the disease.
•ECHOCARDIOGRAM - Aortic enlargement, aortic-septal discontinuity and the aorta overriding the ventricular septum (biventricular aorta) are typical.
•CHEST RADIOGRAPH - Right ventricular enlargement is typical (heart often boot shaped). Aortic arch and knob may be on right side.
•CARDIAC CATHETERIZATION AND ANGIOCARDIOGRAPHY - Typically shows the magnitude of the shunt, morphology of right ventricular outflow tract and if present, anomalous left anterior descending coronary artery.

TRANSPOSITION OF THE GREAT VESSELS
•ECG - Right axis deviation, right atrial enlargement and right ventricular hypertrophy may be seen. Prolonged PR interval or complete heart block may be seen.
•ECHOCARDIOGRAM - Typically shows relative position of great vessels and the shape and internal architecture of the ventricles. Also helpful in identifying commonly associated cardiac defects.
•BLOOD -Polycythemia and decreased O_2 saturation are typical late in the disease.
•CHEST RADIOGRAPH - Large globular heart with increased pulmonary vascular markings is typical.
•CARDIAC CATHETERIZATION - Typically shows the anatomic arrangement of the great vessels.

TRICUSPID REGURGITATION
•ECG - Changes are variable and dependent on etiology.
•CHEST RADIOGRAPH - Marked cardiomegaly, pleural effusion and distention of the azygous vein may be seen. Pulmonary artery and venous hypertension may also be seen.

- •ECHOCARDIOGRAM- Right ventricular diastolic overload pattern with enlarged right ventricle and paradoxical motion of the ventricular septum are typical. With Doppler, can show regurgitant flow from right ventricle into right atrium.
- •CARDIAC CATHETERIZATION - Both right atrial and right ventricular end-diastolic pressures are typically elevated. Right ventriculogram shows extent of regurgitation.

VENTRICULAR SEPTAL DEFECT
- •ECG - Normal in small VSD. Left atrial enlargement and left ventricular hypertrophy are typical with large defects.
- •BLOOD - Polycythemia may be seen.
- •CHEST RADIOGRAPH - Usually normal in small VSD. Left atrial, left ventricular and pulmonary artery enlargement with increased pulmonary vascular markings are typical in large defects.
- •ECHOCARDIOGRAM - Left atrial and left ventricular dilatation, and position of the defect may be seen. Doppler allows calculation of ratio of pulmonary to systemic arterial blood flow.
- •CARDIAC CATHETERIZATION - Typically shows the size and location of the ventricular septal defect. Oxygen saturation step up may be seen at right ventricle level.

COR PULMONALE
- •BLOOD - Arterial blood gas: low PO_2, variable PCO_2 and elevated hematocrit may be seen.
- •CHEST RADIOGRAPH - Enlarged diameter of right and left pulmonary artery may indicate pulmonary hypertension.
- •ECG - Typically shows right atrial enlargement and right ventricular hypertrophy.
- •ECHOCARDIOGRAM with Doppler - Typically shows increased right ventricular size and decreased function.
- •PULMONARY FUNCTION TESTS - Typically show obstructive airway disease.

DRESSLER'S SYNDROME
(POST MYOCARDIAL INFARCTION SYNDROME)
- •ECG - May show ST segment elevations.
- •BLOOD - Elevated ESR, leukocytosis with neutrophil predominance are typical.
- •CHEST RADIOGRAPH - Progressive increase in heart size, transient pleural effusion and pulmonary infiltrate may be seen.
- •ECHOCARDIOGRAM - May demonstrate pericardial effusion.

ENDOCARDITIS (SEE VALVULAR HEART DISEASE)

MYOCARDIAL INFARCTION
- •SERIAL ECGs - May show characteristic changes of acute infarction
- •BLOOD
  - -Creatine Kinase (CK) - may be increased 4-8 hours post infarction and peak at 12-24 hours (may peak earlier if reperfusion occurs), should return to normal by the third day (MB fraction of CK is the best for following progress).
  - -Lactic Dehydrogenase (LDH) - may be increased in 8-12 hours and peak in 3-6 days with elevation continuing up to 10-14 days. Isoenzymes $LDH_1/LDH_2 > 1$, called "flipped LDH" may appear at 12-48 hours (LDH_1 may remain normal).
  - -Serum Aspartate Aminotransferase - may be increased in 8-12 hours, peak at 18-36 hours and return to normal in 3-4 days.
  - -Serum Alpha HBD - may show peak at 4-8 hours with elevation for up to 2 weeks.
  - -Serum MDH - early increase may be seen at 4-6 hours, peak at 24-36 hours and return to normal in approximately 3 days.
  - -Leukocytosis with a slight left shift may be seen.
  - -ESR - may be elevated by the second or third day, peak at 4-5 days and may remain elevated for 2-6 months.
  - -Hyperglycemia is common following acute myocardial infarction.
- •URINE - Glycosuria or myoglobinuria preceding ECG changes may rarely be seen.
- •ECHOCARDIOGRAM - May show regional wall motion abnormality and ventricular dysfunction.
- •RADIONUCLIDE STUDIES
  - -Tc-Pyrophosphate imaging - May show increased uptake (hot spot)·in the area of infarction within 48-72 hours of onset.

PERICARDITIS
- •See Rheumatic Fever, Dressler's Syndrome, Uremia, Bacterial or Viral Infection, and Collagen Vascular Diseases.

ACUTE PERICARDITIS
- •ECG - Serial ECGs may show ST segment elevation (concave upward) in all leads except V_1 and aVR followed by a return of the ST segment to baseline and then T wave inversion.

- BLOOD - WBC often elevated in bacterial pericarditis and Dressler's syndrome, may be normal or low in viral or tuberculous pericarditis. Elevated ESR is common.
- CHEST RADIOGRAPH- Cardiac silhouette may be normal or enlarged (if pericardial effusion is present).
- ECHOCARDIOGRAM - May show pericardial effusion.

<u>PERICARDIAL EFFUSION</u>
- ECG - May show normal or low voltage, atrial arrhythmias, and/or electrical alternans.
- CHEST RADIOGRAPH - May show cardiac enlargement (globular or "water bottle" shape).
- ECHOCARDIOGRAM - Shows echo-free space between the posterior wall of the left ventricle and posterior parietal pericardium and/or between the anterior wall of the right ventricle and anterior parietal pericardium.
- RADIONUCLIDE SCANNING - Tc-labelled albumin aggregates may show abnormal space between heart and adjacent lungs and liver.
- CARDIAC CATHETERIZATION - Diastolic equilibration of ventricular and atrial pressures may be seen in cardiac tamponade.
- PERICARDIOCENTESIS - Usually a transudate. In bacterial, mycotic or parasitic infection the effusion may be an exudate. Hemorrhagic pericarditis (an exudate composed of blood mixed with a fibrinous or suppurative effusion) may be found with tuberculosis, malignancy, anticoagulation or trauma.

<u>CHRONIC CONSTRICTIVE PERICARDITIS</u>
- ECG - Variable changes, atrial arrhythmias are common.
- CHEST RADIOGRAPH/FLUOROSCOPY - May show pericardial calcification.
- CT/MRI - May show thickened/calcified pericardium.
- ECHOCARDIOGRAM/MUGA - Ventricular volume may be normal or decreased with a normal ejection fraction. Pericardial thickening is typical.
- CARDIAC CATHETERIZATION - May show diastolic equilibration of pressure in all chambers of the heart.

RHEUMATIC FEVER   (See RHEUMATOLOGY SECTION)

SHOCK   (See CARDIOGENIC SHOCK)

VALVULAR HEART DISEASE
(See also CONGENITAL HEART DISEASE)

AORTIC REGURGITATION, ACUTE
- •ECHOCARDIOGRAM - Typically shows premature closure of mitral leaflet, may show vegetations or double aortic wall of a dissecting aneurysm. Left ventricle size may be normal or only slightly increased.
- •CARDIAC CATHETERIZATION - Typically shows severity of regurgitation.

AORTIC REGURGITATION, CHRONIC
- •ECG - May show left axis deviation and left ventricular diastolic volume overload.
- •CHEST RADIOGRAPH- Left ventricular enlargement and dilatation of thoracic aorta may be seen.
- •ECHOCARDIOGRAM - May show dilated left ventricle with increased motion of posterior left ventricular wall and interventricular septum. Diastolic flutter of anterior mitral leaflet is often seen. Early changes in left ventricular dysfunction may be seen: increase in end-diastolic and end-systolic diameters and reduced fractional shortening. Doppler echocardiography may show extent of aortic regurgitation.
- •RADIONUCLEOTIDE ANGIOGRAPHY - aortic regurgitation at rest and during graded exercise can be calculated.
- •CARDIAC CATHETERIZATION AND AORTIC ROOT ANGIOGRAPHY- Typically shows extent of regurgitation.

AORTIC STENOSIS
- •CHEST RADIOGRAPH- May show increase in left ventricular size and post stenotic dilatation of the ascending aorta. Calcification of the aortic valve is typically seen with hemodynamically significant aortic stenosis.
- •ECG - Left ventricular hypertrophy and left atrial enlargement are typical in severe stenosis.
- •ECHOCARDIOGRAM - May show dense multiple echoes within the aortic root, and reduced motion of the leaflets. In patients with bicuspid valve, valve cusps are asymmetric with eccentric position in the aortic root. Doppler helps quantify the pressure gradient across the aortic valve.

•CARDIAC CATHETERIZATION - Confirms the gradient, valve area and may show associated lesions including coronary artery disease. Aortic root injection (angiography) can show the number of aortic cusps and aortic insufficiency.

BICUSPID AORTIC VALVE (See AORTIC STENOSIS)

ENDOCARDITIS
•ECG - may show atrioventricular block, arrhythmias or nonspecific ST and T wave changes.
•ECHOCARDIOGRAM - With Doppler may show valve pathology (*ie*, vegetations) or a bulging abscess of the myocardium, valvular ring, or sinus of Valsalva aneurysm. Doppler helps quantify the severity of regurgitation.

BACTERIAL
•BLOOD - Blood cultures are usually positive. Progressive normochromic normocytic anemia with decreased serum iron is common. WBC may be elevated (usually < 15,000/mm^3) with neutrophil predominance. Mono-cytosis may be pronounced and large macrophages may be present on smear. Elevated ESR, cryoglobulins, and rheumatoid factor may be found.

•URINE - Albuminuria and hematuria may be seen.

NONBACTERIAL THROMBOTIC (MARANTIC ENDOCARDITIS)
•ECHOCARDIOGRAM - Involved valve or valve leaflet may show vegetations.

NONBACTERIAL VERRUCOUS ENDOCARDITIS (LIBMAN-SACKS DISEASE)
•See Systemic Lupus Erythematosus
•ECHOCARDIOGRAM - Involved valve or valve leaflet may show vegetations typically smaller than those found in infectious endocarditis.
•BLOOD - Culture negative.

MITRAL STENOSIS
- CHEST RADIOGRAPH - Left atrial enlargement, right ventricular dilatation and prominent pulmonary artery may be seen. Kerley B lines, Kerley A lines and interstitial edema may be seen. Calcification of mitral valves may be seen on fluoroscopy.
- ECG - May show left atrial enlargement (P-mitrale), right ventricular hypertrophy, or atrial fibrillation (usually coarse).
- ECHOCARDIOGRAM - Mitral valve may show thickening, decreased mobility and diminished orifice size.
- CARDIAC CATHETERIZATION - May quantify pulmonary hypertension, pressure gradient across the valve and valve area.

MITRAL VALVE PROLAPSE
- ECG - Premature ventricular beats are common. ST-T changes may be seen.
- 24 hr. AMBULATORY ELECTROCARDIOGRAPHY (HOLTER) - Atrial and ventricular arrhythmias are common.
- CHEST RADIOGRAPH - Minor left atrial enlargement may be seen. Pectus excavatum, straight thoracic spine or scoliosis are sometimes seen.
- ECHOCARDIOGRAM - Prolapsed mitral leaflet may be seen during ventricular systole.
- LEFT VENTRICULOGRAM - Prolapse and scalloped edges of the mitral leaflets may be seen during systole.

MITRAL VALVE REGURGITATION
- ECG - Left atrial enlargement, left ventricular enlargement and atrial fibrillation may be seen.
- CHEST RADIOGRAPH - Cardiomegaly with left ventricular and left atrial enlargement may be seen. Calcification of mitral annulus may be seen in elderly patients.
- ECHOCARDIOGRAM - May show left ventricular volume overload, and enlargement of the left atrium. Underlying cause of the mitral regurgitation, ie, mitral valve prolapse, flail leaflet, ruptured chordae tendineae, vegetations and annular calcification may be seen. Doppler may show high velocity jet in left atrium during systole and helps quantify severity of regurgitation.
- RADIONUCLIDE ANGIOGRAMS - Regurgitant fraction can be calculated.

CARDIOLOGY REFERENCES

ANGINA PECTORIS
1. Silverman, K. J., Grossman, W.: Angina Pectoris: Natural history and strategies for evaluation and management. *N. E. J. M.* 1984; 310:1712-1717.
2. Ellestad, M. H. Stress testing. Principles and Practice, 3rd Ed. Philadelphia, F. A. Davis Co. 1986.
3. Christie, L. G. Jr., Conti, C. R.: Systematic approach to evaluation of angina-like chest pain: Pathophysiology and clinical testing with emphasis on objective documentation of myocardial ischemia. *Am. Heart J.* 1981; 102(5):897-912.

AORTIC DISSECTION
1. Wheat, MW. Jr.: Acute dissecting aneurysms of the aorta: Diagnosis and treatment-1979. *Am. Heart J.* 1980; 99(3):373-387
2. Dalen, J. E., Pape, L. A., Cohn, L. H., Koster, J. K., Collins, J. J. Dissection of the aorta: Pathogenesis, diagnosis and treatment. *Prog. Cardiovasc. Dis.* 1980; 23:237.

CARDIOGENIC SHOCK
1. Wiedermann, H. P., Matthay, M. A., Matthay, R.A.: Cardiovascular-pulmonary monitoring in the intensive care unit: Part I and II. *Chest.* 1984; 85:537-549,656-668.

CARDIOMYOPATHIES
1. Fuster, V., Gersh, B. J., Guiliani, E. R., Tajik, A. J., Brandenburg, R. O., Frye, R. L.: The natural history of idiopathic dilated cardiomyopathy. *Am. J. Cardiol.* 1981; 47:525-531.
2. Wynne, J., Braunwald, E. Cardiomyopathies and myocarditides. In Braunwald, E. (ed). Heart Disease-A Textbook of Cardiovascular Medicine, 3rd Ed. Philadelphia, W. B. Saunders, 1988, pp 1410-1469.
3. Goodwin, J. F., Oakley, C. M.: The Cardiomyopathies. *Br. Heart J.* 1972; 34:545-552.

CONGENITAL HEART DISEASE
1. Perloff, J.K. The clinical recognition of Congenital Heart Disease, 3rd ed. Philadelphia, W. B. Saunders.1987.
2. Roberts W. C. (ed). Adult Congenital Heart Disease. Philadelphia, F.A.Davis, 1986.

ATRIAL SEPTAL DEFECT

1. Feldman, T., Barrow, K. M.: Atrial Septal defects in adults: Diagnosis and management. *Cardiovasc. Med.* 1986; 11:19.

COARCTATION OF AORTA

1. Braunwald, E. (ed). Heart Disease-A Textbook of Cardiovascular Medicine, 3rd Ed. Philadelphia, W. B. Saunders. 1988, pp 994-997.

PATENT DUCTUS ARTERIOSUS

1. Fisher, R. G., Moodie, D. S., Sterba, R., Gill, C. C.: Patent ductus arteriosus in adults-long term follow-up: Nonsurgical versus surgical treatment. *J. Am. Coll. Cardiol.* 1986; 8;280.
2. Braunwald, E. Valvular Heart Disease. In Braunwald, E (ed). Heart Disease, A Textbook of Cardiovascular Medicine. W.B. Saunders Co. 1988.

PULMONARY ATRESIA

1. Perloff, J. K. The Clinical Recognition of Congenital Heart Disease. Philadelphia, W. B. Saunders. 1987, pp 540-552.

TRANSPOSITION OF THE GREAT VESSELS

1. Tonkin IL, Kelly MJ, Bream PR, Elliott LP.: The frontal chest film as a method of suspecting transposition complexes. *Circulation.* 1976; 53;1016.
2. Chin AJ, Yeager SB, Sauders SP, Williams RG, Bierman FZ, Burger BM, Norwood WI, Castaneda AR.: Accuracy of prospective two dimensional echocardiographic evaluation of left ventricular outflow tract in complete transposition of the great arteries. *Am. J. Cardiol.* 1985; 55:759.

VENTRICULAR SEPTAL DEFECT

1. Roberts, W. C. (ed). Adult Congenital Heart Diseases. Philadelphia, F.A. Davis. 1986, pp 409-442.

COR PULMONALE

1. Fishman, A. P. State of the art: Chronic cor pulmonale. *Am. Rev. of Respir. Dis.* 1976; 114:775-793.
2. Braunwald, E. (ed). Heart Disease-A Textbook of Cardiovascular Medicine, 3rd Ed. Philadelphia, W. B. Saunders. 1988, pp 1597-1616.

DRESSLER'S
1. Braunwald, E. (ed). Heart Disease-A Textbook of Cardiovascular Medicine, 3rd Ed. Philadelphia, W. B. Saunders. 1988, pp 1521-1522.

ENDOCARDITIS
1. Kaye, D.: Changing pattern of infective endocarditis. *Am. J. Med.* 1985; 78(6b):157.

MYOCARDIAL INFARCTION
1. Braunwald, E. (ed). Heart Disease-A Textbook of Cardiovascular Medicine, 3rd Ed. Philadelphia, W. B. Saunders. 1988, pp 1222-1313.

PERICARDITIS
1. Spodick, D. H.: Diagnostic electrocardiographic sequences in acute pericarditis: Significance of the PR segment and PR vector changes. *Circulation.* 1973; 48:575.
2. Shabetai, R., Fowler N. O., Guntheroth, W. G.: The hemodynamics of cardiac tamponade and constrictive pericarditis. *Am. J. Cardiol.* 1970; 26:480.
3. Shabetai, R. Progress in cardiac tamponade and constrictive pericarditis. In Yu, P. N., Goodwin, J. F. (ed). Progress in Cardiology. Philadelphia, Lea and Febiger. 1986, pp 87-100.

VALVULAR HEART DISEASE
1. Dalen, J. E., Alpert, J. S. (eds) Valvular Heart Disease, 2nd Ed. Boston, Little, Brown and. 1987.

ACUTE AORTIC REGURGITATION
1. Morganroth, J., Perloff, J. K., Zeldism, S., et al.: Acute severe aortic regurgitation: Pathophysiology, clinical recognition and management. *Ann. Intern. Med.* 1977; 87(2):223-232
2. Masuyama, T, Kodama, K., Kitabatake, A., et al.: Noninvasive evaluation of aortic regurgitation by continuous-wave doppler ECHO. *Circulation.* 1986; 73:460.

AORTIC STENOSIS
1. Gupta, S. C. Aortic Valve Disease, chapter 26. In Barnes, H. V. (ed),Clinical Medicine: Selected problems with pathophysiologic correlations.Chicago, Year Book Medical Publishers. 1988, pp 165-174.

MITRAL VALVE PROLAPSE

1. Abbasi, A. S., DeCristofavo, D., Anabtami, J., Irwin, L.: Mitral Valve Prolapse; Comparative valve of M-mode two dimensional and doppler echocardiography. *J. Am. Coll. Cardiovasc.* 1983: 2;1219-1223.
2. Winkle, R. A., Lopes, M. G., Fitzgerald, J. W.: Arrhythmias in patients with mitral valve prolapse. *Circulation* 1975; 52;73.
3. Wooley, C. F.: The Mitral Valve Prolapse Syndrome. *Hosp. Pract.* 1983; 18(6):163-174.
4. Barlow, J. B., Pocock, W. A.: The mitral valve prolapse enigma-two decades later. *Mod. Concepts Cardiovasc. Dis.* 1984; 53:13-17.

ENDOCRINOLOGY

The number, types and priority of tests ordered must be individualized for each patient, consequently the tests listed for each disease in this chapter are not prioritized and are not exhaustive.

ACROMEGALY
- •BLOOD - Basal human growth hormone (HGH) and Somatomedin C are typically elevated. Growth Hormone Releasing Factor may be elevated in ectopic production syndromes (rare). TRH stimulation test usually shows a paradoxical rise in HGH levels. LHRH stimulation test usually showing a paradoxical rise in HGH levels. Oral glucose tolerance test (100 g) typically shows failure to suppress basal HGH or a paradoxical rise.
- •RADIOGRAPH - Coronal CT scan of pituitary/hypothalamus may show sellar or suprasellar mass.
- •See PITUITARY TUMORS

ADDISON'S DISEASE (See ADRENAL CORTICAL DISEASE, HYPOFUNCTION)

ADRENAL CORTICAL DISEASE
HYPERFUNCTION (CUSHING'S SYNDROME)
- •BLOOD - 8:00 AM cortisol is frequently elevated, 11:00 PM cortisol is usually high suggesting loss of diurnal variation. 8:00 AM cortisol after 1 mg dexamethasone is typically greater than 5 μg/dl.
- •URINE (24 hr.) - urinary free cortisol (UFC) and 17-OH corticosteroids (17-OHCS) are typically elevated if renal function is normal.

(1) ACTH DEPENDENT
Pituitary (Cushing's Disease)
- •BLOOD - Basal DHEA-S is usually elevated and ACTH is usually normal or slightly elevated. CRF stimulation test typically shows hyperresponse of ACTH and/or cortisol.
- •URINE (24 hr) - free cortisol/17-OH corticosteroids are usually elevated. The "low dose" dexamethasone suppression test typically does not show suppression. The "high dose" dexamethasone usually shows >50% decrease from base line values.
- •RADIOGRAPH - Coronal CT of the head is normal in >50% of cases.

(2) ECTOPIC ACTH SYNDROME
- •BLOOD - Basal ACTH is typically elevated, hyperglycemia and hypokalemia are common. CRF stimulation test typically shows no response.
- •URINE (24 hr.) - cortisol/17-OH corticosteroids are usually elevated. "High dose" dexamethasone suppression tests typically shows no suppression.

•RADIOGRAPH - Chest/Abdomen CT Scan - May show tumor of lung, thymus, pancreas or pheochromocytoma.

(3) ACTH INDEPENDENT (ADRENOCORTICAL NEOPLASM)
•BLOOD - The basal ACTH level is usually low or undetectable. The CRF stimulation test typically shows no ACTH/cortisol response.
•URINE - (24 hr) free cortisol/17-OH corticosteroids are usually elevated. The "high dose" dexamethasone suppression test typically shows no response.
•RADIOGRAPH - CT scan of Abdomen - May show an adrenal mass. (Consider presence of pheochromocytoma) See ectopic ACTH.

HYPOFUNCTION (ADDISON'S DISEASE)
PRIMARY ADRENAL FAILURE (End Organ)
   •BLOOD - Basal cortisol may be low and ACTH elevated. ACTH stimulation test (1 Hour) shows poor or no cortisol response, aldosterone response poor.

SECONDARY ADRENAL FAILURE (Pituitary)
   •BLOOD - Basal cortisol and ACTH may be low. ACTH stimulation test (1 Hour) - Shows poor or no cortisol response. Aldosterone response is typically normal.
   •RADIOGRAPH - Coronal CT Scan of pituitary/hypothalamus may show space occupying lesion.

ADRENAL TUMORS
   •BLOOD - Basal testosterone, DHEA's are typically elevated in androgen producing tumors. Catecholamines may be elevated in pheochromocytoma. Aldosterone may be elevated and renin suppressed in primary aldosteronism (see detail below). Estrogen levels may be elevated in feminizing adrenal tumors, (17-OH progesterone, 11-deoxycortisol, pregnenalone may also be elevated).
   •URINE - VMA and metanephrines are typically elevated in pheochromocytoma. 24 hour urinary free cortisol and 17-OH corticosteroids typically may be elevated in Cushings. 17-ketosteroids are typically elevated in androgen producing tumors.
   •RADIOGRAPH - Abdominal CT or MRI may aid in defining the anatomy and the mass.

ALDOSTERONISM
PRIMARY
- BLOOD - Basal hypokalemia, metabolic alkalosis, elevated aldosterone, and low plasma renin activity (PRA) are typical. Provocative PRA may show inadequate response to upright posture and sodium depletion. Aldosterone does not suppress with supine posture and sodium loading.
- URINE (24hr.) - Elevated aldosterone and potassium are typical.

ADRENAL ADENOMA (CONN'S SYNDROME)
- BLOOD - Basal 18-OH Corticosterone is usually increased. Stimulation - Aldosterone falls in most cases with upright posture. Suppression - Captopril test usually shows no decrease in serum aldosterone. Selective adrenal vein sampling - unilateral elevation of aldosterone may be seen.
- RADIOGRAPH - Abdominal CT Scan - Unilateral adrenal enlargement may be seen. Iodocholesterol scanning may show unilateral uptake in tumor.

IDIOPATHIC ADRENAL HYPERPLASIA
- BLOOD - Basal - 18 OH Corticosterone is usually not elevated. Provocative - Increase in aldosterone with upright posture. Suppression - Captopril usually shows a decrease in serum aldosterone. Selective sampling - No lateralization of aldosterone production is typical.
- RADIOGRAPH - CT Scan Abdomen - Normal or bilateral enlargement of adrenals may be seen. Iodocholesterol scanning may show bilateral uptake.

SECONDARY
GENERAL
- BLOOD - Aldosterone and renin are typically elevated. Sodium may be low.

BARTTER'S SYNDROME
- BLOOD - Potassium decreased with pH, aldosterone, renin, and chloride typically elevated.
- URINE - Urine potassium and chloride levels are usually elevated.

AMENORRHEA (FEMALE HYPOGONADISM)
PRIMARY AMENORRHEA
•BLOOD - Karyotype may be XO, XY, XX, or mosaic patterns.
  -LH, FSH, E_2, T_3RU, T_3, TSH and Prolactin may be abnormal
    depending on the underlying pathology.

SECONDARY AMENORRHEA
•BLOOD - Basal ßeta-HCG is positive in pregnancy. LH, FSH, E_2,
  T_3RU, T_3, TSH and Prolactin may be abnormal depending on the
  underlying pathology.
•RADIOGRAPH - Coronal CT Scan of the pituitary/hypothalamus may
  show tumor etiology.

AMIODORONE INDUCED THYROID DISEASE
•BLOOD (clinically euthyroid subjects) -T_4, RT_3, TSH may show dose
  dependent transient increase, T_3 may be decreased.
  TRH Stimulation test - Hyperreactive TSH response may be seen.
•NUCLEAR MEDICINE - RAIU may be decreased.

HYPERTHYROIDISM
•BLOOD - T_3 and Free T_3 concentrations are typically increased.

HYPOTHYROIDISM
•BLOOD - Antimicrosomal antibodies commonly positive, elevated
  TSH.

ANDROGEN DEFICIENCY (MALE HYPOGONADISM)
PRIMARY GONADAL FAILURE
•BLOOD - Karyotype may show 47 XXY = Klinefelter's Syndrome or
  mosaic pattern. LH, FSH are typically elevated and testosterone
  (free) is typically decreased.
  - HCG stimulation usually shows no increase in testosterone level.
•Sperm Count - Decreased to azospermia.
•Buccal Smear - positive sex chromatin (Barr Body) may occur in
  Klinefelter's Syndrome.

SECONDARY GONADAL FAILURE
•BLOOD - LH, FSH and testosterone may be low and prolactin may
  be elevated (see hyperprolactinemia). Ferritin level is typically
  elevated in hemochromatosis. LHRH Stimulation test typically

shows no response with a pituitary lesion. Delayed and/or diminished response is consistent with a hypothalamic lesion
•RADIOGRAPH - Coronal CT Scan of the pituitary/hypothalamus may show a mass.

BONE DISEASE (METABOLIC)
•BLOOD -
Alkaline Phosphatase is typically low in hypophosphatasia, typically high in Paget's disease, hyperparathyroidism, fracture healing, prepubertal and pubertal growth.

Calcium - Is typically elevated in hyperparathyroidism, may be elevated in malignancy and rarely in hyperthyroidism. Typically low in hypoparathyroidism and osteomalacia.

Phosphate - Usually elevated in hypoparathyroidism. Typically low in hyperparathyroidism and osteomalacia.

Osteocalcium (bone GLA protein) (reflects bone turnover) - Is typically low during glucocorticoid treatment and senile osteoporosis. Typically high in primary hyperparathyroidism, renal osteodystrophy.

Paget's disease and hyperthyroidism.

Vitamin D metabolites
25 (OH) Vit. D - Typically elevated in Vit. D intoxication and usually low in osteomalacia, and ricketts.
1-25 (OH)$_2$ Vit. D - Typically high in hyperparathyroidism, sarcoid and some hematologic malignancies. Usually low in hypoparathyroidism and renal failure.

•URINE (24 hr.) (see Parathyroid disease)
Hydroxyproline - Low or normal is typical in simple osteoporosis (senile). Typically high in Paget's disease, hyperparathyroidism, hyperthyroidism, puberty, skeletal metastasis, fracture, burn patients, psoriasis and acromegaly.

•RADIOGRAPH - Plain films - may show typical lesions of specific conditions.Photon absorptiometry (Measures bone mineral density) - May suggest demineralization.

•NUCLEAR MEDICINE - Bone scanning may show uptake in metastasis, fracture, and Paget's lesions.

CARCINOID SYNDROME
•URINE (24 hr) - 5-HIAA - typically elevated.
False negative 5-HIAA results may occur in pyridoxal-phosphate deficiency, intestinal obstruction, small intestine resection and phenothiazine ingestion.

False positive 5-HIAA results may be seen with the ingestion of
bananas, walnuts and glycerol guiacolate.
5-Hydroxytryptophan may be elevated in gastric carcinoid.
•RADIOGRAPH - CT Scan of Chest - may show bronchial lesion if
present and upper GI series, barium enema may localize a
primary lesion in the gut.

CONGENITAL ADRENAL HYPERPLASIA
<u>21-Hydroxylase deficiency</u> (95% of cases reported)
•BLOOD - 17-OH progesterone and ACTH are usually elevated.
Cortisol and aldosterone are typically suppressed. ACTH
stimulation test usually shows exaggerated 17-OH progesterone
response in late onset congenital adrenal hyperplasia.
•URINE (24 hr) - Urinary free cortisol and 17-OH corticosteroids are
typically depressed. Pregnanetriol and 17 ketosteroids are
typically elevated.

11-HYDROXYLASE DEFICIENCY
•BLOOD - 11 deoxycortisol, deoxycorticosterone and ACTH are
usually elevated. Serum cortisol may be low.
•URINE - 17 ketosteroids are typically elevated.

3-ß -HYDROXYSTEROID DEHYDROGENASE DEFICIENCY
•BLOOD - DHEA and DHEA-S are typically elevated. Cortisol and
aldosterone are usually decreased.
•Urine - 17 ketosteroids are typically elevated.

CUSHINGS SYNDROME (See ADRENAL DISEASE, HYPERFUNCTION)

DIABETES
<u>INSIPIDUS</u>
•BLOOD - Hyperosmolarity is typical.
•URINE - Compared to simultaneous blood draw is hyposmolar
•Water Deprivation Test - Urine osmolarity typically increases to
normal = primary polydipsia. Urine volume is high and osmolarity
remains low, reverses with ADH = central diabetes insipidus.
Urine volume high/osmolarity remains low and no response to
ADH = Nephrogenic diabetes insipidus.

<u>MELLITUS</u>
- BLOOD - Fasting blood sugar greater than 140 mg/dl on two separate samples. HbA1C typically elevated. Low Insulin/C-peptide is typical in insulin dependent diabetes mellitus (Type 1). Normal to elevated insulin level is typical of non-insulin dependent diabetes mellitus (Type II). Oral Glucose Tolerance Test -Blood sugar is typically greater than 200mg/dl x 2 from 0-2 hours after 75g glucose load.
- URINE - Glucosuria occurs when plasma glucose is greater than renal resorption threshold. Ketonuria may be seen.

EMPTY SELLA SYNDROME
- BLOOD - Occasional elevation of prolactin is seen. Releasing factor stimulation tests are usually normal.
- RADIOGRAPHY - Lateral skull film may show enlarged sella. Coronal CT Scan of head - Typically shows CSF density only in sella area.

GALACTORRHEA
- Breast secretion typically stains positive for fat.
- BLOOD - Basal prolactin level may be elevated (see prolactinoma). Growth hormone is rarely elevated (see acromegaly). T3RU, T4 may be decreased with elevated TSH (see primary Hypothyroidism) or T4 increased in hyperthyroidism.
- RADIOGRAPHY - Coronal CT Scan of Sella - may show pituitary tumor *if* prolactin is elevated.
- Visual Fields - May show bitemporal hemianopsia with pituitary tumor.

GRAVES' DISEASE   (SEE THYROTOXICOSIS)

GROWTH HORMONE DEFICIENCY
- BLOOD - Basal - Growth Hormone (HGH) is frequently normal but may be low or non-measurable. Somatomedin C is frequently normal but may be low. Stimulation - Fails to elicit a HGH response with at least two tests: GRF, insulin tolerance, arginine, L-DOPA, exercise.
- RADIOGRAPH - Coronal CT Scan of Head - may show a pituitary/hypothalamic lesion.

GYNECOMASTIA
- BLOOD - Estrogen may be increased with testicular tumor, bronchogenic carcinoma, true hermaphrodite and some adrenal tumors. T_3RU, T_4 and T_3RIA are typically elevated in hyperthyroidism. Liver function tests may be abnormal in liver disease (cirrhosis).
- Buccal Smear - Positive sex chromatin (Barr Body) may be seen and requires karyotype for confirmation of genetic syndromes such as Kleinfelter's, etc.
- RADIOGRAPH - Mammogram may demonstrate a mass in breast cancer.

HIRSUTISM
- BLOOD - Free testosterone level may be elevated due to adrenal or ovarian overproduction or increased peripheral conversion of androstenedione to testosterone. Prolactin may be elevated. DHEA-S may be elevated in adrenal overproduction. LH/FSH ratio typically increased in polycystic ovary syndrome. 17-OH progesterone typically elevated in congenital adrenal hyperplasia (21-OH deficiency).
  Suppression - Overnight dexamethasone suppression test may be abnormal with Cushing's.
  Stimulation - Elevated 17-OH progesterone after ACTH in late onset 21-OH deficiency may be seen.
- URINE (24 hr.) 17-OH corticosteroids and free cortisol are typically elevated in Cushing's. 17 ketosteroids usually markedly elevated in adrenal cancer.
- RADIOGRAPH - adrenal vein sampling may lateralize testosterone secretion. CT Scan of adrenals may reveal adrenal mass. Pelvic Ultrasound may show polycystic ovaries or ovarian mass.

HYPOADRENALISM (See ADRENAL CORTICAL DISEASE)

HYPOGLYCEMIA
- BLOOD - Plasma glucose is typically less than 45 mg/dl in true hypoglycemia. Insulin/glucose ratio typically greater than 0.3 in insulin mediated hypoglycemia. C-peptide is typically elevated if excess endogenous insulin secretion and undetectable or low in factitious hypoglycemia.

-Non Suppressible Insulin-like Activity (NSILA) may be detectable when associated with large mesenchymal tumors. ACTH stimulation test is typically abnormal in primary adrenal failure. A 72 hour fast usually produces hypoglycemia due to insulinoma.
•RADIOGRAPH -May show pancreatic tumor in insulinoma.

HYPOGONADISM (See AMENORRHEA and ANDROGEN DEFICIENCY)

HYPOPITUITARISM (See PITUITARY DISEASE, FUNCTIONAL)

HYPORENINEMIC HYPOALDOSTERONISM
•BLOOD - Basal - Aldosterone level is typically decreased, hyperkalemia, mild renal failure and hyperglycemia may be seen. Renin does not increase following stimulation.

IMPOTENCE (See ANDROGEN DEFICIENCY)

KALLMAN'S SYNDROME (HYPOGONADOTROPHIC HYPOGONADISM)
•BLOOD - LH, FSH, testosterone are typically low.
LHRH Test- LH/FSH levels typically increase.

KLINEFELTER'S SYNDROME (See ANDROGEN DEFICIENCY)

LITHIUM TOXICITY
•BLOOD - T_4, T_3, RT_3 may be decreased. TSH and serum osmolarity may be increased.
•URINE - Specific gravity and osmolarity are typically low (see Nephrogenic Diabetes Insipidus).

OSTEOMALACIA (See BONE DISEASE, METABOLIC)

OSTEOPENIA (See BONE DISEASE, METABOLIC)

OSTEOPOROSIS (See Bone Disease, Metabolic)
•BLOOD - Usually normal calcium and thyroid function.
•RADIOGRAPH - Bone mineral densitometry is variable (usually low compared to age/sex norms).

OVARIAN TUMORS
- •BLOOD - Androgens may be elevated especially testosterone.
  Estrogens typically elevated (LH/FSH suppressed) in granulosa
  theca cell tumors. HCG typically elevated in choriocarcinoma.
  Thyroxine typically elevated in struma ovarii (see
  Hyperthyroidism).
- •URINE (24 hr.) - 17 ketosteroids may be markedly elevated in
  association with malignant adrenal-like tumors.
  -5-HIAA may be elevated in carcinoid.
- •RADIOGRAPH - Pelvic ultrasound may reveal ovarian mass.

PAGET'S DISEASE (See BONE DISEASE, METABOLIC)

PANCREATIC TUMORS
ISLET CELL TUMORS
GASTRINOMA (ZOLLINGER-ELLISON SYNDROME)
- •BLOOD: Basal - gastrin level may be markedly elevated.
  Calcium/Secretin stimulation test usually produces an
  increase in gastrin levels.
- •GASTRIC ANALYSIS - Gastric acid production is typically
  elevated.
- •RADIOGRAPH - Abdominal CT Scan - may show pancreatic
  mass. Upper GI Series - May show peptic ulcer disease.

GLUCAGONOMA
- •BLOOD - Moderate hyperglycemia and anemia may be seen.
  Glucagon level is typically elevated. Tolbutamide
  stimulation test typically shows an increase in glucagon
  (rarely a necessary test).
- •RADIOGRAPH - Abdominal CT Scan may show pancreatic
  mass.

INSULINOMA - See Hypoglycemia.

PANCREATIC POLYPEPTIDE PRODUCING TUMORS (PPoma)
- •BLOOD - Basal - Pancreatic polypeptide level is typically
  elevated. Provocative meal usually results in an elevated
  pancreatic polypeptide level.
- •RADIOGRAPH - Abdominal CT Scan - May show a pancreatic
  mass.

SOMATOSTATINOMA
- •BLOOD Basal - Glucose usually moderately elevated and insulin/glucagon is typically low. Somatostatin level is typically elevated as are the liver function tests with metastasis.
- •GASTRIC ANALYSIS - Typically shows hypochlorhydria.
- •RADIOGRAPH - Gall stones often present on oral cholecystogram and gall bladder ultrasound. Abdominal CT Scan - May show pancreatic mass.

VIPoma (PANCREATIC CHOLERA SYNDROME)
- •BLOOD - Usually shows hypokalemia and metabolic acidosis. Vasoactive Intestinal Polypeptide (VIP) is typically elevated. Hypercalcemia, hypomagnesemia, hyperglycemia may occur.
- •GASTRIC ANALYSIS - Usually shows hypochlorhydria.
- •RADIOGRAPH - Abdominal CT Scan - May show pancreatic mass.

PANHYPOPITUITARISM - See PITUITARY DISEASE, FUNCTIONAL

PARATHYROID DISEASE
PRIMARY HYPERPARATHYROIDISM
- •BLOOD - Calcium, parathyroid hormone, 1,25 $(OH)_2$ Vit. D, chloride are typically elevated. Bicarbonate, phosphate are usually decreased. T_3RIA and angiotension converting enzyme are typically normal.
- •URINE (24 hr.) - Calcium, cAMP and phosphate are typically elevated.
- •RADIOGRAPH - Ultrasound may identify gland enlargement/adenoma.
- •NUCLEAR MEDICINE - Tc-Thallium subtraction scan may show uptake in adenoma.
SECONDARY HYPERPARATHYROIDISM
- •BLOOD - Calcium (ionized) typically low and phosphate may be elevated. 25 (OH) Vit. D and 1,25 $(OH)_2$ Vit. D may be low. BUN/creatinine are frequently elevated along with PTH (N-terminal).
- •URINE - Typically elevated cAMP and decreased creatinine clearance is common.

<u>HYPOPARATHYROIDISM</u>
PRIMARY HYPOPARATHYROIDISM
- •BLOOD - Hypocalcemia, hyperphosphatemia are typical and
25 (OH) Vit. D is usually normal. Parathyroid hormone levels
and 1,25 (OH)$_2$ Vit. D are typically decreased. Parathyroid
antibodies may be positive in Type I polyendocrine failure.
Ferritin and Iron are typically elevated in hemochromatosis.
- •URINE (24 hr.)- cAMP and calcium excretion are usually low with
increased cAMP after exogenous PTH.
PSEUDOHYPOPARATHYROIDISM
Type I
- •BLOOD - PTH is typically elevated, 25 (OH) Vit. D is usually
normal and 1,25 (OH)$_2$ Vit. D is typically decreased.
- •URINE - cAMP is typically decreased with no change after
  exogenous PTH.
Type II
- •BLOOD - PTH is typically elevated, 25 (OH) Vit. D is usually
normal, 1,25 (OH)$_2$ Vit. D is typically decreased.
- •URINE - cAMP typically elevated and increases further with
exogenous PTH.

PHEOCHROMOCYTOMA - See ADRENAL TUMORS

PITUITARY DISEASE
<u>HYPERFUNCTION</u> - See Acromegaly, Cushing's Disease,
Prolactinoma
- •BLOOD - Basal LH, FSH, LH/FSH elevation with normal or low
testosterone may be seen in gonadotropin tumor (see also
Androgen Deficiency). TSH is typically elevated - with
elevated thyroxine level in TSH secreting pituitary tumor (see
also Hyperthyroidism).
- •RADIOGRAPH - Coronal CT Scan of head - may reveal sellar
enlargement, tumor or suprasellar extension.

<u>HYPOFUNCTION</u>
ANTERIOR
- •BLOOD - Basal - Low levels of ACTH, TSH, LH, FSH, GH, or
PRL with correspondingly low levels of cortisol, thyroxine,
sex steroids (low sperm counts/amenorrhea) or
somatomedin-C may be seen.

Tests of pituitary-adrenal reserve.
- CRF test typically shows no ACTH/cortisol response.
- Insulin/Metyrapone test typically shows no ACTH/cortisol response.
- 1 Hour ACTH stimulation test often shows no cortisol response with a normal aldosterone response (secondary hypoadrenalism).
- Prolonged ACTH stimulation test typically shows recovery of cortisol and 17-OH corticosteroid secretion.
- TRH test typically shows no increase in TSH or prolactin.
- LHRH test typically shows no increase in LH/FSH response.
- Insulin tolerance test usually shows no GH, cortisol or prolactin response.
- L-DOPA, L-arginine exercise stimulation tests usually show no significant HGH response.

POLYENDOCRINE FAILURE SYNDROME
• BLOOD -HLA-B8 is seen with increased frequency.

POSTPARTUM PITUITARY NECROSIS (SHEEHAN'S SYNDROME)
• BLOOD - Basal - Usually shows low prolactin, T_4/TSH, E_2/LH-FSH, cortisol/ACTH (One or more may be affected).
- CRF test typically shows no increase in ACTH/cortisol.
- 1 hour ACTH simulation test early in course may be normal. Late in the course there may be an increase in cortisol.
- TRH test usually shows no increase inTSH or prolactin.
- LHRH test usually shows no increase in LH/FSH response.

PROLACTINOMA
• BLOOD - Basal - Prolactin level is usually greater than 100 ng/ml. T_3Ru, T_4, TSH, BUN, creatinine are typically normal. TRH Stimulation typically shows no prolactin response.
• RADIOGRAPH - Coronal CT Scan of sella/hypothalamus may show mass.
• Visual Field Testing - May show bitemporal hemianopsia.

PSEUDOHERMAPHRODITISM

FEMALE (Male phenotype with ovaries)
- •BLOOD - Typically shows XX karyotype. Androgen overproduction is typical (See Congenital Adrenal Hyperplasia).

MALE (Female phenotype with testes)
- •BLOOD - Typically shows XY Karyotype. Testosterone is usually normal, high or low with variable gonadotropin levels depending on pathophysiology.

STRUMA OVARII - See THYROID DISEASE and OVARIAN TUMORS

TESTICULAR TUMOR
- •BLOOD - Basal - HCG typically is elevated in germ cell tumors. Alpha-fetoprotein is typically elevated in yolk sac tumors. Carcinoembryonic Antigen (CEA) may be elevated in some teratomas. Estradiol is usually elevated in feminizing tumors suppressed with LH/FSH.
- •RADIOGRAPH - Scrotal ultrasound may reveal subtle abnormalities suggesting a tumor mass.

THYROID DISEASE

HYPERTHYROXINEMIA (With THYROTOXICOSIS)
- •BLOOD - Liver function tests and calcium may be elevated. WBC may be decreased with relative lymphocytosis. Total and free thyroxine usually elevated. Total and free triiodothyronine are usually elevated (especially in nodular hyperthyroidism).TSH is typically suppressed to undetectable levels except in TSH secreting pituitary tumors. Thyroglobulin is typically elevated except in L-thyroxine and/or T_3 ingestion. Thyroid stimulating Immunoglobulin is usually elevated in Grave's disease. HCG activity is typically elevated in trophoblastic mediated disease. Antimicrosomal and Antithyroglobulin antibodies are usually present in autoimmune mediated thyroid disease. ESR may be elevated in subacute thyroiditis (painful). TSH stimulation test typically shows no rise in TSH.
- •NUCLEAR MEDICINE
Radioactive Iodine Uptake (RAIU) -Typically increased in Grave's, nodular toxic goiter (uninodular/multi-nodular) and HCG or TSH mediated disease. Typically decreased in subacute thyroiditis, painless thyroiditis, L- thyroxine ingestion, ectopic thyroid

hormone production (lingular goiter, struma ovarii, metastatic cancer), iodine induced or treated hyperthyroidism.
-Thyroid Scan - Diffuse uptake is typical in Grave's disease Solitary nodule with remainder of gland suppressed = Plummer's disease. Patchy uptake typical in toxic multinodular goiter. Whole body scan may reveal ectopic hormone production site.
•RADIOGRAPH - Orbital CT Scan may show thickened extraocular muscles in Grave's disease.

HYPERTHYROXINEMIA (Without THYROTOXICOSIS)
Familial Dysalbuminemic Hyperthyroxinemia (FDH)
•BLOOD - Total T_4 typically elevated, specific protein electrophoresis is typically abnormal. Free T_4, TSH and Free T_3 are typically normal. TRH stimulation test is typically normal.
•NUCLEAR MEDICINE - RAIU is typically normal.

HYPOTHYROIDISM
•BLOOD - Total and Free T_4 are typically decreased, TBG concentration may be increased. Total and Free T_3 are usually normal in early stages. TSH is usually elevated in primary thyroid failure and normal or low in secondary or tertiary disease. Prolactin, CPK, LDH, SGOT, catecholamines and their metabolites may be elevated. Antimicrosomal, antithyroglobulin antibodies are typically positive in Hashimoto's. Anemia - normochromic, microcytic, macrocytic (may be B_{12} mediated) may be seen. Cholesterol and triglyceride may be elevated. Sodium and glucose may be low.
•RADIOGRAPH - Coronal CT Scan may show sellar enlargement.

THYROID DISEASE, STRUCTURAL
THYROID ENLARGEMENT (GOITER)
•BLOOD - T_3RU, T_4, T_3RIA, TSH - are typically normal. Antimicrosomal, antithyroglobulin antibodies, if positive suggests autoimmune etiology.Thyrocalcitonin - is usually elevated in medullary carcinoma (usually solitary nodule). Calcium/Pentagastrin stimulation test may show an increase in calcitonin in the presence of C-cell hyperplasia.
•RADIOGRAPH- Ultrasound may differentiate solid versus cyst.
•PATHOLOGY - Fine needle aspiration cytology may delineate malignancy vs. benign lesion.

TURNER'S SYNDROME
- •BLOOD - Classic karyotype 45 XO. LH/FSH are typically increased and E_2 is typically low. Positive antithyroid antibodies with T_4 increased or decreased may be seen with associated autoimmune thyroid disease.
- •BUCCAL SMEAR - Typically negative for sex chromatin (Barr Body).

ZOLLINGER-ELLISON SYNDROME - (See PANCREATIC TUMORS)

ENDOCRINE REFERENCES

ACROMEGALY
1. Ho, K. Y., Evans, W. S., Thormer, M. O.: Disorders of prolactin and growth hormone production. *Clinics Endo. Metab.* 1985(14);1:1-32.
2 Kao, P. C., Abbound, C. F., Zimmerman, D.: Somatomedin-C: An index of growth hormone activity. *Mayo. Clinic Proc.* 1986; 61:908-909.

ADRENAL CORTICAL DISEASE
1. Bondy, P. K.: Disorders of the adrenal cortex. In Williams, Textbook of Endocrinology, 7th Ed. Philadelphia, W.B. Saunders Comp. 1985, pp 816-891.
2. Copeland, P. M.: The incidentally Discovered Adrenal Mass. *Ann. Intern. Med.* 1983; 98:940-945.

ALDOSTERONISM
1. Drury, P. L.: Disorders of Mineralcorticoid Activity. *Clinics Endo. Metabol.* 1985(14); 1:175-202.

AMIODARONE AND IODINE INDUCED THYROID DISEASE
1. Braverman, L. E., Burger, A. G.: Iodine induced changes of thyroid function. In Werner, The Thyroid Gland, 5th Ed. Philadelphia, J. B. Lippincott. 1986.

BONE DISEASE METABOLIC
1. Aurbach, G. D., Marx, S. J., Spiegel, A. M.: Metabolic bone disease. In Williams, Textbook of Endocrinology, 7th Ed. Philadelphia, W. B. Saunders Comp. 1985, pp 1218-1255.
2. Lukert , B. P., et al.: Serum osteocalcium is increased in patients with hypothyroidism and decreased in patients receiving Glucocorticoids. *J. Clinic. Endo. Med.* 1986; 62:1056-1058.

CONGENITAL ADRENAL HYPERPLASIA
1. Bongiovanni, A.: In James, H. T. (ed), The Endocrine function of the Human Adrenal Cortex. New York, Academic Press. 1978, p 265.

FEMALE GONADAL DYSFUNCTION
1. Morris, D. V., Adams, J., Jacobs, H. S.: The Investigation of female Gonadal Dysfunction. *Clinic Endo. Metabol.* 1985(14); 1:125-143.

HIRSUTISM
1. Rittmaster, R. S., Loriaux, D. L.: *Ann. Intern. Med.* 1987; 106:95-107.

HYPOGLYCEMIA
1. Nelson, R. L.: Hypoglycemia: Fact or fiction. *Mayo. Clin. Proc.* 1985; 60:844-850.

PANCREATIC ISLET CELL TUMORS
1. Krejs, G. J.: Non-insulin secreting tumors of the pancreatic islets. In Williams, Textbook of Endocrinology, 7th Ed. Philadelphia, W. B. Saunders Comp. 1985, pp 1301-1309.

PARATHYROID
1. Levine, M. A.: Laboratory investigation of disorders of the parathyroid glands. *Clinics Endo. Metabol.* 1985(14); 1:257-272.

PITUITARY ANTERIOR
1. Daughaday, W. H.: In Williams, Textbook of Endocrinology, 7th Ed. Philadelphia, W. B. Saunders Comp. 1985, pp 568-613.

PROLACTINOMA
1. Ho, K. Y., Evans, W. S., Thormer, M. O.: Disorders of prolactin and growth hormone production. *Clinics Endo. Metabol.* 1985(14); 1:1-32.

THYROID DISEASE
1. Ingbar, Branerman: In Werner, The Thyroid Gland, 5th Ed. Philadelphia, J. B. Lippincott. 1986.
2. Laderson, P. W.: Diseases of the Thyroid Gland. *Clinics Endo. Metabol.* 1985(14); 1:145-174.

GASTROENTEROLOGY

The number, types and priority of tests ordered must be individualized for each patient, consequently the tests listed for each disease in this chapter are not prioritized and are not exhaustive.

ABSCESS   (PANCREATIC)
•BLOOD - Elevated WBC is common. Blood cultures may be positive.
•CT SCAN - Cystic structure. May see air bubbles in retroperitoneum.
•ENDOSOCPIC RETROGRADE CHOLANGIOPANCREATOGRAPHY
   - Dye may fill cyst.

APPENDICITIS
•URINE - RBC's may be present.
•BLOOD - Elevated WBC (leukocytosis with PMN predominance).
   Electrolyte changes may be consistent with vomiting.
•RADIOGRAPHY
   Abdominal Flat Plate - Small bowel loops with air fluid levels,
      occasionally a gas-filled appendix or fecalith present.
   CXR - Occasionally shows right basal pneumonitis and/or
      atelectasis.

BOWEL OBSTRUCTION
PYLORIC
•RADIOGRAPHY
   Abdominal Flat Plate - Gastric distention is seen.
   Upper GI Series- Scarring or complete blockage at the pylorus is
      typical.
•ESOPHAGOGASTRODUODENOSCOPY - Scarring or complete
   blockage at the pylorus may be seen.

SMALL BOWEL
•RADIOGRAPHY - Abdominal flat plate - Air fluid levels in small bowel
   with dilated loops are typical.

LARGE BOWEL
•RADIOGRAPHY
   Abdominal Flat Plate- Dilated loops of colon, may or may not have
      small bowel dilatation.
   Barium Enema - Barium stops at level of obstruction.
•COLONOSCOPY - May visualize actual obstruction.

CARBOHYDRATE INTOLERANCE
•BLOOD - Increased serum transaminases and lactic acidosis may be
   seen in fructose intolerance.
•LACTOSE TOLERANCE TEST - May be abnormal in lactose
   intolerance.

•HYDROGEN BREATH TEST - May be abnormal in lactose intolerance.
•CHROMATOGRAPHY - Urine fructose is seen.
•SMALL BOWEL BIOPSY WITH MUCOSAL ASSAYS - May show enzymatic deficiencies.

CHOLECYSTITIS
•See Choledocholithiasis.
•BLOOD - elevated WBC, AST, ALT, alkaline phosphatase, bilirubin and GGT may be seen.
•RADIONUCLIDE IMAGING (e.g. HIDA, PIPIDA, OR DISIDA) - Typically shows non-filling of the gallbladder.

CHOLEDOCHOLITHIASIS
•BLOOD - Elevated bilirubin, alkaline phosphatase and GGT may be seen.
•RADIOGRAPHY
   CT/Ultrasound - dilated common bile duct may be visualized with obstruction, stone may also be visualized.
   Endoscopic Retrograde Cholangiopancreatography - non-filling or obstruction of the common bile duct is seen (this procedure may allow stone removal).
   Percutaneous Transhepatic Cholangiogram - Dilated common bile duct may be visualized.
•DUODENAL ASPIRATE - May show cholesterol crystals.

CHOLELITHIASIS
•RADIOGRAPHY
   Ultrasound, CT, Endoscopic Retrograde Cholangiopancreatography, oral cholecystogram may visualize stones.

CROHN'S DISEASE (SEE INFLAMMATORY BOWEL DISEASE)

CIRRHOSIS
GENERAL
•BLOOD - Elevated AST and ALT are typical, occasionally alkaline phosphatase and bilirubin are elevated, macrocytic anemia, prolonged PT time, hypo-albuminemia, hypergammaglobulinemia, elevated ammonia level (especially in those with hepatic encephalopathy) may be seen. Decreased magnesium,

phosphate and sodium and alpha-1-antitrypsin. (COPD often an associated abnormality) may be seen.

ALCOHOLIC
- BIOPSY - Liver: steatosis, polymorphonuclear infiltrate, fibrosis and micronodular cirrhosis, Mallory bodies are typical, with concomitant hepatitis.

VIRAL HEPATITIS
- BLOOD - HB surface and/or HB core antigen are often positive (may have associated Delta Virus).
- BIOPSY - Liver: lymphocytic inflammation in the periportal and parenchymal areas, fibrosis, and macronodular pattern, special stains may reveal viral particles.

PRIMARY BILIARY CIRRHOSIS
- BLOOD - Elevated alkaline phosphatase and cholesterol are typical. May find abnormalities consistent with rheumatologic disease, ie. antimitochondrial antibodies, and/or antinuclear antibodies
- BIOPSY- Liver: Destructive lesions of the bile ductules, lymphocyte infiltrate, fibrosis and cirrhosis are typical.

HEMOCHROMATOSIS
- BLOOD - Elevated serum iron and ferritin with increased transferrin saturation are typical.
- URINE - Urinary iron excretion is increased by chelating agent Deferoxamine.
- BIOPSY - Liver: Marked iron deposition in hepatocytes (quantitative iron measurement may be indicated).

WILSON'S DISEASE (HEPATO-LENTICULAR DEGENERATION)
- BLOOD - Low ceruloplasmin, hemolytic anemia and elevated transaminase are typical.
- URINE - Elevated copper excretion may be seen.
- BIOPSY - Liver: elevated copper concentration from dried liver sample, pattern consistent with chronic active hepatitis and cirrhosis.
- SLIT LAMP EYE EXAM - Descemet's membrane may demonstrate Kayser-Fleischer ring.
- MAGNETIC RESONANCE IMAGING - May show necrosis in basal ganglia and white matter of the brain.

COLON CARCINOMA
- •BLOOD- Microcytic anemia, elevated AST, alkaline phosphatase, bilirubin (especially with hepatic metastasis), and CEA may be seen.
- •STOOL - Typically heme positive.
- •RADIOGRAPHY

  Barium Enema - Mass or constrictive lesion may be seen.

  CT Scan - Liver metastasis, adenopathy, or primary mass may be seen.
- •ENDOSCOPY

  Colonoscopy with Biopsy - Mass may be ulcerated or friable, biopsy usually shows adenocarcinoma.

  Proctosigmoidoscopy - Mass lesion may be seen.

CRIGLER-NAJJAR SYNDROME
- •BLOOD - Elevated unconjugated bilirubin with normal liver function tests.
- •PHENOBARBITAL TRIAL - Type I: no response

  Type II: reduces bilirubin to 4-6 mg%.
- •BIOPSY - Liver: Histology usually normal but glucuronyl transferase deficiency is present.

DIARRHEA (CHRONIC)
Key tests depend on clinical presentation.
- •BLOOD - Micro / macrocytic anemia and electrolyte abnormalities (ie. decreased potassium), elevation of 5 -HIAA (carcinoid), serotonin, gastrin (hormone secreting tumors) and PT, and decreased cholesterol, calcium and albumin may be seen.
- •URINE - 5-HIAA may be elevated in carcinoid.
- •STOOL - Quantitative fecal fat elevated, ova and parasites, fasting 24 hour stool volume (> 500cc in secretory diarrhea), high stool PH (possible laxative abuse), stool osmolality > plasma (osmotic diarrhea).
- •d-XYLOSE ABSORPTION TEST - Test will be abnormal if mucosal disease.
- •RADIOGRAPHY - Barium enema with small bowel follow through may show abnormality. Skeletal films may reveal decreased bone density.
- •BIOPSY - Rectal: May be abnormal in inflammatory bowel disease.
- •BENTIROMIDE URINARY EXCRETION TEST - Typically abnormal in pancreatic insufficiency.

DUBIN-JOHNSON SYNDROME
- BLOOD - Elevated conjugated bilirubin.
- URINE - Corproporphyrin ratio I/III may be increased (increased 1, decreased 2).
- BIOPSY - Liver: Is often pigmented (brown/black).
- BSP - Delayed rise after 90-120 minutes may be seen.

DYSPHAGIA
- RADIOGRAPHY
  - CXR - If malignant etiology may demonstrate hilar mass, if achalasia may demonstrate air fluid levels in the esophagus.
  - Barium Swallow - If malignant etiology may demonstrate a mass lesion, if achalasia a stricture may be seen.
  - Nuclear Medicine Scan - may show delayed transit through the esophagus.
- MANOMETRY - If achalasia, high distal esophageal pressure without relaxation may be seen, or simultaneous contraction may be seen.
- EGD - Mass, strictures, or esophagitis may be seen.

ESOPHAGEAL SPASM
- RADIOGRAPHY - Upper GI Series- corkscrew pattern may be seen.
  - Nuclear Medicine Scan - May show delayed transit through the esophagus.
- MANOMETRY - Symptomatic pain associated with pressure change.

ESOPHAGEAL VARICES
- BARIUM SWALLOW - Serpeginous defects may be seen.
- EGD - Distended veins in esophagus may be visualized.

FAMILIAL POLYPOSIS
- BLOOD - Mild decrease in hemoglobin and hematocrit may be seen.
- STOOL - Heme positive is typical.
- COLONOSCOPY with BIOPSY- Many polyps, histologically adenomas may be seen.
- BARIUM ENEMA- multiple polyps are typical.

GARDNER'S SYNDROME
- STOOL - Typically heme positive.
- RADIOGRAPHY - Mandible and maxilla endosteoid osteomas, unerupted teeth and dense bone in place of trabeculae, long bone osteomas and thick, irregular densities may be seen.
  - Barium Enema - Multiple polyps are typical.

GAY BOWEL SYNDROME
- BLOOD - VDRL and HIV may be positive.
- STOOL - Cultures for: Amebiasis, *Shigella, Chlamydia trachomata, Gonorrhea* , Herpes Simplex Virus, Condyloma *accuminatum, and Isospora deli* may be positive.
- PROCTOSIGMOIDOSCOPY - Fissures, perirectal abscesses, proctitis (may necessitate biopsy and culture) perianal ulcers are often seen.

GILBERT'S SYNDROME
- BLOOD - Elevated unconjugated bilirubin (especially with prolonged fasting) normal liver function tests.
- PHENOBARBITAL TRIAL - Bilirubin may return to normal values.

GLYCOGEN STORAGE DISEASES
von GIERKE (GLUCOSE 6-PHOSPHATASE DEFICIENCY)
- Blood glucose may be very low.
- Liver enzymes may be normal or slightly increased.
- Lactic acidosis may be present.
- Hyperlipidemia - Cholesterol and triglycerides may be markedly elevated.
- Hyperuricemia may be present.

GLUCOSE 6-PHOSPHATASE MICROSOMAL TRANSLOCASE DEFICIENCY
- Laboratory Studies: Same as for Glucose 6-phoshatase deficiency.
- Neutropenia frequently seen.

CORI (DEBRANCHER ENZYME DEFICIENCY)
- Typically normal Lactate.
- Typically normal Uric acid.
- Increased Cholesterol may be seen.
- Increased Triglyceride may be seen.
- Increased AST may be seen.

HERS (HEPATIC PHOSPHORYLASE DEFICIENCY)
- Hyperlipidemia may be present.

<u>McCARDLE (MUSCLE PHOSPHORYLASE DEFICIENCY)</u>
•Increased CPK may be seen.
•Ischemic exercise test with deficient lactate production may be seen.
•Myoglobinuria may be present.

<u>POMPE (LYSOSOMAL ALPHA-GLUCOSIDASE DEFICIENCY)</u>
•Increased CPK may be present.
•No hypoglycemia usually seen.

<u>ANDERSON (BRANCHER ENZYME DEFICIENCY)</u>
•No hypoglycemia usually seen.

HEMOCHROMATOSIS (SEE CIRRRHOSIS)

HEPATITIS (VIRAL)
ACUTE HEPATITIS (B, AND NON-A/NON-B)
•BLOOD - Lymphopenia and neutropenia may be seen with the onset
  of fever, then elevated WBC with macrocytosis and lymphocytosis
  (may also see plasma cells and atypical lymphocytes). ESR
  (especially during the icteric period), ALT, AST, alkaline
  phosphatase, bilirubin, transaminase and aldolase may be
  increased. Hemolytic anemia may be present and haptoglobulin
  may be decreased.
•URINE - Bilirubinuria (usually occurs before elevated serum bilirubin)
  may be seen.

<u>HEPATITIS A</u>
•SEROLOGY - Anti-HAV IgM elevation occurs early, anti HAV-IgG
  elevation after the acute period (may remain detectable for life).

<u>HEPATITIS B</u>
•SEROLOGY
  - HBsAg elevation (first indicator of infection, and remains elevated
  through the acute period).
  - HBeAg follows HBsAg in appearance and disappears prior to
  HBsAg clearing (associated with the highly infectious state).
  -Anti-HBc-Total - appears after HBsAg and HBeAg but before their
  respective antibodies. If measured during the serologic window it
  may be the only serologic marker present. The IgM fraction is only
  present during acute disease, the IgG fraction may persist for
  years.

-Anti-HBe - associated with decreased infectivity, helps to confirm recent acute infection when associated with anti-HBc and negative HBsAg and anti-HBs absent.

-Anti-HBs - associated with recovery and immunity to HBV (when no HBsAg is detectable). In fulminant hepatitis there may be anti-HBs coexistent with low antigen titers.

CHRONIC HEPATITIS (HEPATITIS B)
•BLOOD - After the acute period, ALT and AST decreases toward normal, HBsAg usually remains high with continued presence of HBeAg, and increased gamma globulin.
•BIOPSY - Liver: May reveal cirrhosis with lymphocytic inflammation in the periportal and parenchymal areas, fibrosis, macronodular pattern, special stains may reveal intracellular viral particles.

HEPATOCELLULAR CARCINOMA
•BLOOD - Alpha Fetoprotein elevation and increased hematocrit may be seen
•RADIOGRAPHY
  CT/Ultrasound - Mass may be visualized.
  Gallium Scan - Positive uptake in tumor.
  Angiography - Neovascularization of mass.
•BIOPSY - Liver: may see tumor cells recognizable as hepatocytic.

INFLAMMATORY BOWEL DISEASE
GENERAL
•BLOOD - Elevated WBC, ESR, platelets, AST, alkaline phosphatase, and bilirubin may be seen (especially when pericholangitis and/or sclerosing cholangitis are associated). Micro/macrocytic anemia may be present.

CROHN'S DISEASE
•RADIOGRAPHY
  Abdominal Flat Plate - Thickened loops of small bowel, and obstruction with perforation (free air) may be seen.
  Barium Enema - Strictures (string sign), fistula, colitis may be seen
  Upper GI with Small Bowel follow through - Strictures (string sign), fistula and separation of loops.

•ENDOSCOPY

Proctoscopy - Rectal involvement with anal sparing may be seen.
Colonoscopy with biopsy - Colon may or may not be involved, if
involved, lesions are patchy with apthous ulcerations of bowel.
Biopsy may show granulomas.
Endoscopic Gastroduodenoscopy - aphthous or serpinginous
ulcerations (more frequent in duodenum) may be seen.

ULCERATIVE COLITITIS
•RADIOGRAPHY

Abdominal Flat Plate - May show distended large bowel (toxic
megacolon).
Barium Enema - Ulcerations, distension and "Lead Pipe"
appearance of colon may be seen.
•ENDOSCOPY

Proctoscopy - May show ulcerations in rectum.
Colonoscopy with Biopsy - colon involvement with ulcers,
pseudopolyps and adenocarcinoma with longstanding
disease.

JUVENILE POLYPOSIS
•STOOL - May be heme positive.
•BARIUM ENEMA - Single or multiple polyps may be seen.
•COLONOSCOPY with BIOPSY - Small, pedunculated polyps,
histologically hamartomas (rarely adenocarcinoma).
•ESOPHAGO-GASTRO DUODENOSCOPY - may reveal polyps
(usually not done).

MACROAMYLASEMIA
•BLOOD - Elevated amylase, abnormal amylase electrophoretic
pattern.

MALABSORPTION   (SEE DIARRHEA, CHRONIC)

MALLORY WEISS TEAR
•UPPER GI SERIES - Esophageal linear tears may be seen with
severe disease.
•ESOPHAGO-GASTRO DUODENOSCOPY- Tears may be visualized
within the first 24 hours.

MESENTERIC VASCULAR OCCLUSION

- •BLOOD - Elevated hemoglobin and hematocrit, leukocytosis (often > 20,000), elevated lipase, amylase and phosphate, metabolic acidosis (late finding) may be seen.
- •STOOL - Typically heme positive.
- •RADIOGRAPHY

  Abdominal Flat Plate - Early may show complete absence of air; later generalized distention. "Thumb-printing": bowel wall thickening and gas in bowel wall may be seen.

  Angiography - Narrowing, spasm or occlusion of the branches or origins of the celiac, superior mesenteric artery, inferior mesenteric artery and their branches may be seen.

  Barium Enema - While not recommended, if done may show narrowing, spasm and "Thumb-printing." In time, there may be loss of haustra or narrowing of the bowel.

  Small Bowel Series - Edema, spasm, blunted folds, separation of loops, "picket fence" appearance are typical.
- •EXPLORATORY LAPAROTOMY - May be required for diagnosis.

PANCREATIC CARCINOMA

- •BLOOD - Amylase and lipase may be slightly elevated in early stages. Glucose tolerance test may show diabetic curve (some will develop overt diabetes). Elevated CEA, bilirubin (mostly direct), alkaline phosphatase, and leucine aminopeptidase (rarely used clinically) may be seen.
- •RADIOGRAPHY

  CT/Ultrasound - May visualize a mass or show dilated bile duct or pancreatic duct.

  ENDOSCOPIC RETROGRADE CHOLANGIOPANCREATOGRAPHY -

  Obstruction of pancreatic or bile duct may be seen.

  Radioisotope scanning of pancreas (Selenium) - May demonstrate pancreatic duct obstruction (rarely used clinically).
- •BIOPSY - Open or CT directed needle aspirate may show adenocarcinoma.
- •TRIOLIEN 131-I TEST - May demonstrate pancreatic duct obstruction (rarely used clinically).

PANCREATITIS

ACUTE

- BLOOD - Lipase/amylase elevation (amylase is the first to rise but also the first to fall) (see macroamylasemia). Decreased calcium (usually in severe cases 1-9 days after onset), amylase/creatinine ratio is increased, elevated trypsin, mild elevation of WBC and hematocrit may be seen.
- URINE - Amylase may be elevated (if no renal disease).
- ULTRASOUND - Pancreatic enlargement with decreased density may be seen.
- CT SCAN- Pancreatic enlargement and decreased density with peripancreatic edema may be seen.

CHRONIC

- BLOOD - Amylase and lipase increase after administration of pancreozymin and secretin, fasting serum lipase increased in 10% of patients, abnormal oral glucose tolerance test may be seen.
- STOOL - Steatorrhea.
- RADIOGRAPHY
  Abdominal Flat Plate - may show diffuse, stippled pancreatic calcification (observed in approximately 30% of patients).
- ERCP - Pancreatic duct is irregularly strictured and dilated ("chain of lakes").
- BENTIROMIDE (CHYMEX) TEST - decreased urine level of Para-amino Benzoic Acid.

PEPTIC ULCER

- BLOOD - Micro/macrocytic anemia, elevated calcium, elevated gastrin.
- UPPER GI SERIES - Ulcer crater, (immobile pocket of barium), deformed duodenal bulb may be seen with old ulcer. Benign ulcers usually extend beyond the lumen of the stomach,have a smooth bed and often exhibit a radiolucent line (of normal mucosa). Malignant ulcers usually do not extend beyond the lumen of the stomach, have an irregular base and the ulcer crater is often eccentrically located.
- ESOPHAGO-GASTRO DUODENOSCOPY with BIOPSY - An erythematous crater with edema, benign ulcers have a smooth mound with normal rugae radiating to the ulcer base. Malignant ulcers usually show an irregular base and are eccentrically located.

PERITONITIS
- •BLOOD - Elevated WBC is typical, and blood cultures may be positive.
- •PARACENTESIS - Leukocytosis with increased neutrophils, low pH, elevated lactate may be seen, gram stain and culture for bacteria usually polymicrobial.
- •RADIOGRAPHY
  Barium Enema: May show diffuse ileus.
  Abdominal Flat Plate: May show free air in peritoneal cavity.

SPONTANEOUS BACTERIAL PERITONITIS
- •BLOOD - Increased WBC, blood cultures may be positive.
- •Paracentesis - Usually one organism, no evidence of bowel perforation.

PEUTZ-JEGHERS SYNDROME
- •BLOOD - Decreased hemoglobin and hematocrit may be seen.
- •STOOL - May be heme positive.
- •BARIUM ENEMA - Multiple hamartomas (polyps) may be seen.
- •COLONOSCOPY with BIOPSY - Polyps, histologically hamartomas.

PSEUDOCYST, (PANCREATIC)
- •BLOOD - Elevated direct bilirubin and alkaline phosphatase may be seen with biliary obstruction, elevated amylase and lipase and increased fasting blood sugar may be seen.
- •STOOL - Increased fecal fat.
- •SECTETIN-PANCREOZYMIN STIMULATION TEST- Duodenal contents usually have decreased bicarbonate.
- •ULTRASOUND - may see cystic lesion.
- •CT - cystic lesion.

ROTER'S SYNDROME
- •BLOOD - Mild chronic conjugated hyperbilirubinemia.
- •ORAL CHOLECTSTOGRAM - Typically normal.

ULCERATIVE COLITIS (SEE INFLAMMATORY BOWEL DISEASE)

VIPOMA
- •BLOOD - Decreased potassium and chloride and increased calcium and PTH, metabolic acidosis (with watery diarrhea) and elevated VIP are typical.

GASTROENTEROLOGY REFERENCES

ABCESS (PANCREATIC)
1. Ranson, J.H.C., Balthazar, E., Caccavale R. et al.: Computed
   tomography and the prediction of pancreatic abcess in acute
   pancreatitis. *Ann Surg* 201:656-663.

APPENDICITIS
1. Condon, R.E. Appendicitis. In Sabiston (ed): Textbood of surgery,
   13th Ed. Philadelpha, W.B. Saunders Co. 1986 pp 967-982.

BOWEL OBSTRUCTION
1. Cohn, I. Intestinal obstruction. In Berk (ed): Gastroenterology,
   4th Ed., vol 3. Philadelphia, W.B. Saunders Co. 1985, pp 2056-2080.

CARBOHYDRATE INTOLERANCE
1. Spiro, H.M. Carbohydrate intolerance. In Spiro (Ed): Clinical
   Gastroenterology, 3rd Ed. Philadelphia, W.B. Saunders Co. 1983
   pp 576-84.

CHOLECYSTITIS
1. Weissman, H.S.: Spectrum of 99 m-Te-IDA cholescintigraphic
   patterns in acute cholecystitis. *Radiol* 1981; 138:167.

CHOLEDOCHOLITHIASIS
1. Berk, J.E., Meshkinpour, H., Schapiro, M., et al. Choledocholithiasis.
   In Berk (ed): Gastroenterology, 4th Ed. , vol 3. Philadelphia, W.B.
   Saunders Co. 1985, pp 3693-3712.

CHOLELITHIASIS
1. Crade, M.: Surgical and pathological correlation of cholecystography.
   Am. J. Radiol 1978; 131:227-229.

CIRRHOSIS
1. Rankin, J.G., Orrego-Matte H., Deschenes J., et al.: Alcoholic liver
   disease: The problem of diagnosis. *Alcoholism* 1978; 2:327-338.
2. Kaplelman, Schaffner, F.: The natural history of primary biliary
   cirrhosis. *Semin Liver Dis* 1981; 1:273-281.
3. Halliday J.W., Cowishaw J.C., Russo AM et al. Serum ferritin in the
   diagnosis of hemochromatosis. *Lancet* 1977; 1:621-624.

COLON CARCINOMA
1. Winawer, S.J., Sherlock, P. Malignant neoplasms of the small and large intestine. In Sleisenger and Fordtran (Eds): Gastrointestinal diseases, 5th Ed. Philadelphia, W.B. Saunders Co. 1983, pp 1220-1259.

CRIGLER-NAJJAR SYNDROME
1. Billing, B., Bilirubin metabolism. In Schiff (Ed): Diseases of the liver, 5th Ed. Philadelphia, J.B. Lippincott 1982, pp 349-378.

DIARRHEA
1. Read, N.W., Krejs, G.J., Read, M.G. et al.: Chronic diarrhea of unknown etiology. *Gastroenterol* 1980; 78:264-271.

DUBIN - JOHNSON SYNDROME
1. Billing, B. Bilirubin metabolism. In Schiff (Ed): Diseases of the liver, 5th Ed. Philadelphia, J.B. Lippincott 1982, pp 349-378.

DYSPHAGIA
1. Pope, CE. Motor disorders. In Sleisenger and Fordtran (Eds): Gastrointestinal Diseases, 5th Ed. Philadelphia, W.B. Saunders Co. 1983 pp 424-448.

ESOPHAGEAL SPASM
1. Bennett, J.R.: Esophageal spasm-- as clinicians see it. *J Clin Gastroenterol* 1985; 7:463-466.

ESOPHAGEAL VARICES
1. Waldram, R., Nunnerley, H., Davis, M., et al.: Detection and grading of esophageal varices by fiberoptic endoscopy and barium swallow with and without Buscopan. *Clin Radiol* 1977; 28:137-141.

FAMILIAL POLYPOSIS
1. Bowland, C.R., Kim, Y.S. Colonic polyps and the gastrointestinal polyposis syndrome. In Sleisenger and Fordtran (Eds): Gastrointestinal diseases, 5th Ed. Philadelphia, W.B. Saunders Co. 1983 pp 1196-1219.

GARDENER'S SYNDROME
1. Bowland C.R., Kim, Y.S. Colonic polyps and the gastrointestinal polyposis syndrome. In Sleisenger and Fordtran (Eds): Gastrointestinal diseases, 5th Ed. Philadelphia, W.B. Saunders Co. 1983, pp 1196-1219.

GAY BOWEL SYNDROME
1. Smith, P.D., Lane, H.C., Gill, V.J ,et al.: Intestinal infections in patients with AIDS. *Ann Intern Med* 1988; 108:328-333.

GILBERT'S SYNDROME
1. Orolicsanyi, L., Fevery, J., Billing, B.H., et al.: How should mild, isolated unconjugated hyperbilirubinemia be investigated? *Sem Liver Dis* 1983; 3:65-72.

GLYCOGEN STORAGE DISEASE
1. Sharp, H.L. Inherited disorders with metabolic hepatic dysfunctions. In Berk (ed): Gastroenterology, 4th ED. Philadelphia, W.B.Saunders Co. 1985, pp 3250-3252.

HEPATITIS (VIRAL)
1. Hoofnagle, J.H. Schafer DF.: Serologic markers of hepatitis B virus infection. *Seminars in liver disease* 1986;6:1-10
2. Mijch, A.M. Gust I.D.: Clinical, serologic and epidemiologic aspects of hepatitis A virus. *Seminars in liver disease* 1986;6:42-45.

HEPATOCELLULAR CARCINOMA
1. DiBisceglia, A.M., Rustgi V.K., Hoofingle, J.H. et al.: Hepatocellular Carcinoma. *Ann Intern Med* 1988; 108:390-401.

INFLAMMATORY BOWEL DISEASE
1. Donaldson, R.M. Crohn's disease. In Sleisenger and Fordtran (Eds): Gastrointestinal diseases, 5th Ed. Philadelphia, W.B. Saunders Co. 1983 pp 1088-1121.
2. Cello, J.P.. Ulcerative colitis. In Sleisenger and Fordtran (Eds): Gastrointestinal diseases, 5th Ed. Philadelphia, W.B. Saunders Co. 1983 pp 1122-1168.

JUVENILE POLYPOSIS
1. Bowland, C.R., Kim, Y.S. Colonic polyps and the gastrointestinal polyposis syndrome. In Sleisenger and Fordtran (Eds): Gastrointestinal diseases, 5th Ed. Philadelphia, W.B. Saunders Co. 1983 pp 1196-1219.

MACROAMYLASEMIA
1. Berk J.E. Macroamylasemia. In Berk (ed): Gastroenterology, 4th ED. Philadelphia, W.B.Saunders Co. 1985, pp 4072-4080.

MALLORY-WEISS
1. Graham, D.Y., Schwartz, J.T.: The spectrum of the Mallory-Weiss tear. *Medicine* 1977; 57:307-318.

MESENTERIC VASCULAR OCCLUSION
1. Grendell, J.H., Ockner, R.K. Vascular diseases of the bowel. In Sleisenger and Fordtran (Eds): Gastrointestinal diseases, 5th Ed. Philadelphia, W.B. Saunders Co. 1983 pp 1543-1568.

PANCREATIC CARCINOMA
1. Van Dyke, J.A., Stanley, R.J., Berland, L.L.: Pancreatic imaging. *Am Intern Med* 1985; 102:212-217.

PANCREATITIS
1. Geokas, M.C., Baltaxe, H.A., Banks, PA, et al. Acute pancreatitis.: *Ann Intern. Med* 1985; 103:86-100.

PERITONITIS
1. Diethelm, A.G. The acute abdomen. In Sabiston (Ed): Textbook of Surgery, 13th Ed. Philadelphia, W.B. Saunders Co. 1986 pp 790-809.

PEPTIC ULCER
1. Dooley, C.P., Larson, A.W., Stace, N.H. et al.: Double-contrast barium meal and upper gastrointestinal endoscopy. *Ann Intern Med* 1984; 101:538-545.

PEUTZ-JEGHERS SYNDROME
1. Bowland, C.R., Kim, Y.S. Colonic polyps and the gastrointestinal polyposis syndrome. In Sleisenger and Fordtran (Eds): Gastrointestinal diseases, 5th Ed. Philadelphia, W.B. Saunders Co. 1983, pp 1196-1219.

PSEUDOCYST (PANCREATIC)
1. Barkin, J,S,, Goldberg, H., Bradley EL. Cysts and pseudocysts of the pancreas. In Berk (ed): Gastroenterology, 4th Ed. , vol 6. Philadelphia, W.B. Saunders Co. 1985, pp 4145-4151.

ROTOR'S SYNDROME
1. Wolkoff, A.W., Wolpert, E., Pascasia, F.N., et al. Rotor's syndrome, a distinct inheritable pathophysiologic entity.: *Am J Med* 1976; 60:173-179.

VIPOMA

1. Morrissey, J.F. Clinical approach to diagnostic endoscopy in patients with upper gastrointestinal bleeding.: *Dig Dis Sci* 1981; 26 (suppl):6s-11s.

HEMATOLOGY
ONCOLOGY

The number, types and priority of tests ordered must be individualized for each patient, consequently the tests listed for each disease in this chapter are not prioritized and are not exhaustive.

ANEMIAS

ANEMIA OF CHRONIC DISEASE
- •BLOOD - Hemoglobin, hematocrit, iron and total iron binding capacity are typically decreased. Ferritin is normal to increased, typically a normocytic normochromic on blood smear, reticulocyte normal or decreased.
- •BONE MARROW ASPIRATION AND BIOPSY - Iron is typically present in macrophages.

APLASTIC ANEMIA
- •BLOOD - Decreased hemoglobin, hematocrit, reticulocyte count, platelets and leukocytes may be seen. Usually normochromic, normocytic anemia by indices and blood smear.
- •BONE MARROW ASPIRATION AND BIOPSY - Typically hypoplastic.

AUTOIMMUNE HEMOLYTIC ANEMIA
- •BLOOD - Hemoglobin and hematocrit are usually decreased. Positive direct. Coombs is typical. Reticulocyte count, indirect bilirubin and LDH are usually increased, MCV variable, platelet count normal or decreased, spherocytes typically present on smear, haptoglobin normal or decreased.

GLUCOSE-6-PHOSPHATE DEHYDROGENASE (G-6-PD) DEFICIENCY
- •URINE - Hemosiderin or free hemoglobin may be present.
- •BLOOD - Hemoglobin and hematocrit are decreased, Heinz bodies may be seen in RBC's. Reticulocytes are typically increased. Serum indirect bilirubin and lactate dehydrogenase may be elevated, haptoglobin may be decreased,free hemoglobin may be elevated. G-6-PD activitiy of RBC's is reduced. (It is important to note that G-6-PD activity may appear normal during or soon after a hemolytic crisis if the majority of the deficient cells have been eliminated).

HEREDITARY ELLIPTOCYTOSIS
- •BLOOD - Elevated reticulocyte count, normochromic normocytic anemia, increased elliptocytes, decreased haptoglobin, elevated bilirubin and LDH are typical.

HEREDITARY SPHEROCYTOSIS
- •BLOOD - Decreased hemoglobin and hematocrit, elevated reticulocytes, normal MCV and MCHC are typical. Serum indirect

bilirubin and LDH may be elevated. Spherocytes typically present on peripheral smear. Coombs test should be negative. Serum haptoglobin may be depressed. Osmotic fragility of RBC's is typically increased.

IRON DEFICIENCY
- BLOOD - Decreased hemoglobin and hematocrit, MCV, MCHC, and MCH, increased or normal platelet count, hypochromic microcytic RBCs on smear, normal or decreased reticulocyte count. Decreased ferritin and iron and increased total iron binding capacity are typical.
- BONE MARROW ASPIRATION AND BIOPSY - Absent iron by stain.

MEGALOBLASTIC ANEMIA
- URINE - Schilling test assesses intrinsic factor production and ileal absorbtion of B_{12}, and may aid in differentiating pernicious anemia from other forms of B_{12} deficiency (ie. inadequate intake).
- BLOOD - Increased MCV, decreased reticulocyte count, normal platelet count or decreased, oval macrocytes and hyper-segmented PMN's on smear, leukopenia (severe cases), decreased vitamin B_{12} and/or folic acid, increased LDH and indirect bilirubin, and decreased hemoglobin and hematocrit are typical.
- BONE MARROW ASPIRATION AND BIOPSY - Megaloblastic changes.

PAROXYSMAL NOCTURNAL HEMOGLOBINURIA
- URINE - May contain hemosiderin or free hemoglobin.
- BLOOD - Hemoglobin and hematocrit are typically decreased, often leukopenia and/or thrombocytopenia. Reticulocytes are usually elevated. MCV is variable. Serum indirect bilirubin and LDH may be elevated. Haptoglobin may be decreased. Sucrose hemolysis test should be positive. Diagnosis is confirmed by a positive Ham acid hemolysis test. Red cell acetylcholinesterase activity is typically low.
- BONE MARROW ASPIRATION AND BIOPSY - Erythroid hyperplasia is often present, but cellularity is variable. All three cell lines may be hypoplastic. Iron is often absent.

SICKLE CELL B-THALASSEMIA
- BLOOD - Decreased hemoglobin and hematocrit, increased sickled RBCs, hypochromic microcytic anemia, anisocytosis, poikilocytosis,target cells, fragmented RBC's, Howell-Jolly Bodies, increased WBC with left shift, and increased reticulocyte count are typical.
- Hemoglobin Electrophoresis - HbS (β6 GLU --> VAL), elevated HbA$_2$ and fetal hemoglobin are typical.

SICKLE CELL/HEMOGLOBIN C
- BLOOD - Decreased hemoglobin and hematocrit, sickled cells on blood smear, poikilocytosis, target cells, HbC crystals in RBCs, and elevated reticulocyte count are typical.
- Sickle-Cell Screening Test (Na metabisulfite sickle cell prep) - Usually shows sickling.
- Hemoglobin Electrophoresis - HbC (β6 GLU --> LYS) and HbS (β6 GLU --> VAL) are typical.

SICKLE CELL DISEASE
- BLOOD - Decreased hemoglobin and hematocrit, elevated platelet count sickled cells on blood smear, normocytic normochromic, Howell-Jolly bodies,fragmented RBCs, and elevated reticulocyte count are typical. Increased indirect bilirubin,and increased RBC lactate dehydrogenase may be seen.
- Sickle-Cell Screening Test (Na metabisulfite sickle cell prep) - Typically shows sickling.
- Hemoglobin Electrophoresis - HbSS (β6 GLU --> VAL), Homozygous are typical.

SICKLE CELL TRAIT
- BLOOD - Smear may show few target cells.
- Sickle-Cell Screening Test (Na metabisulfite sickle cell prep) - May show small amount of sickling.
- Hemoglobin Electrophoresis - Hb-AS (35-40% Hb-S, 55-60% Hb-A).

SIDEROBLASTIC ANEMIA
- BLOOD - Elevated serum iron and transferrin saturation, normal or low MCV, dimorphic RBCs with basophilic stippling (sometimes hypochromic), and normal or decreased reticulocyte and platelet counts are typical.

•BONE MARROW ASPIRATION and BIOPSY - Ring sideroblasts are
  typically seen.

BLADDER CANCER
•URINE - Gross or microscopic hematuria.
•URINE CYTOLOGY - From bladder wash, catheterization or voided
  urine may visualize neoplastic cells.
•Cystoscopic Evaluation with Tumor Biopsy may show:
    -transitional cell carcinoma (more common among cigarette
      smokers and workers in the dye, chemical, and certain rubber
      industries),
    -squamous cell carcinoma (more common in patients with chronic
      infestation of *schistosoma haematobium*).
•IVP - May show unilateral or bilateral urethral obstruction with
  hydronephrosis. A filling defect or decrease in bladder
  distensibility may be seen.

BLEEDING DISORDERS
HEMOPHILIA A - DEFICIENCY OF FACTOR VIII
•BLOOD - Activated partial thromboplastin time (PTT) prolonged
  (corrected by adsorbed plasma). Bleeding time and PT are
  typically normal. Decreased Factor VIII:C, normal factor VIII
  antigen, and normal factor VIII:ristocetin cofactor are typical.

FACTOR XI
•BLOOD - Prolonged PTT, and normal PT and bleeding time are
  characteristic, Factor XI is typically decreased.

FACTOR XII DEFICIENCY (HAGEMAN FACTOR)
•BLOOD - Elevated PTT, normal PT, and no correction with serum
  from an established case of Factor XII deficiency are typical.

FACTOR XIII (FIBRIN-STABILIZING FACTOR) DEFICIENCY
•BLOOD - Decreased Factor XIII level, and normal routine tests of
  blood coagulation and platelet function are typical.
•LABORATORY DIAGNOSIS consists of demonstrating that a fibrin
  clot, made by recalcifying the patient's plasma sample, dissolves
  overnight at room temperature in 5 M urea or 1% monochloracetic
  acid is characteristic.

<u>HEMOPHILIA B - DEFICIENCY OF FACTOR IX</u>
•BLOOD - PTT prolonged (in mild forms). PTT is typically corrected by
  normal serum, but not by adsorbed plasma. Prothrombin time and
  bleeding time are typically normal. Factor IX is characteristically
  decreased.

<u>VITAMIN K DEFICIENCY</u>
•BLOOD - Elevated PT and PTT correctable with vitamin K in vivo are
  typical.PT and PTT typically corrects after the addition of normal
  serum in vitro. Bleeding time and fibrinogen are usually normal.

<u>VITAMIN K DEPENDENT FACTORS</u>

   <u>FACTOR IX DEFICIENCY</u> - Covered under Hemophilia B.

   <u>FACTOR VII DEFICIENCY</u>
   •BLOOD - Increased PT, normal bleeding time, and normal PTT
    are typical.
   •Confirmation is aided by an inability to correct the patient's PT
    with plasma from a person known to have Factor VII deficiency.

   <u>FACTOR X (STUART-PROWER) DEFICIENCY</u>
   •BLOOD - Increased PT and PTT and normal bleeding time are
    typical.
   •PT and PTT should correct with normal serum, but not with
    adsorbed plasma.

   <u>AFIBRINOGENEMIA</u>
   •BLOOD - Prolonged PT, PTT and bleeding time, and decreased
    fibrinogen are typical.

   <u>PROTHROMBIN DEFICIENCY</u>
   •BLOOD - Decreased prothrombin, prolonged PT and PTT, normal
    bleeding time, thrombin time and fibrinogen level are typical.
   •Typically uncorrectable with serum or adsorbed plasma.

<u>VON WILLEBRAND'S DISEASE</u>
•BLOOD - Prolonged bleeding time, abnormal ristocetin-induced
  platelet aggregation, normal PT, and normal platelet count and
  morphology are typical. The following may vary depending on the
  subtype: FVIII/VWF decreased, FVIII : C decreased, FVIII : antigen
  decreased, FVIII ristocetin cofactor decreased.

114

COLD AGGLUTININ SYNDROME
- •BLOOD - Usually negative direct Coombs using polyspecific antisera. Positive direct Coombs using monospecific C_3 antisera, negative direct Coombs using monospecific IgG antisera, and cold agglutinin titer of 100 or greater at 4° C are typical. Blood on smear may have RBC clumps (often an artifactually high MCH and MCHC due to clumps), elevated reticulocyte count, and atypical lymphocytes (when associated with mononucleosis).
- •MONOSPOT - may be positive when associated with infectious mononucleosis.
- •SERUM PROTEIN ELECTROPHORESIS - occasionally shows a monoclonal spike.

DISSEMINATED INTRAVASCULAR COAGULATION
- •BLOOD - Thrombocytopenia, prolonged PT and PTT, decreased fibrinogen, and elevated fibrin degradation products are typical.

ESSENTIAL THROMBOCYTOSIS
- •BLOOD - Elevated platelet count ($>1\times10^6/\mu L$). On smear: platelets are often large and hypogranular, platelet aggregation may be abnormal in response to ADP, epinephrine, or collagen.
- •BONE MARROW ASPIRATION AND BIOPSY - The number of hyperploid megakaryocytes, and increased reticulin may be seen.

EVANS' SYNDROME (COMBINED AUTOIMMUNE HEMOLYTIC ANEMIA AND THROMBOCYTOPENIA)
- •BLOOD - Hemoglobin and hematocrit are normal to decreased. Thrombocytopenia, spherocytosis, red cell fragmentation, polychromasia, elevated reticulocyte count, positive direct Coombs, elevated indirect bilirubin and LDH, decreased haptoglobin and elevated anti-platelet immunoglobulins may be seen.

HEMOCHROMATOSIS
- •URINE - Increased urinary iron excretion by chelating agent deferoxamine is typical.
- •BLOOD - Elevated serum iron and ferritin with increased transferrin saturation are typical
- •BIOPSY - Liver: Siderosis, cirrhosis (quantitative iron measurement of iron from sample may be indicated) are typical.

HEMOLYTIC UREMIC SYNDROME (GASSER'S SYNDROME)
- •URINE - Proteinuria and micro or gross hematuria are typical.
- •BLOOD - Decreased platelet count, schistocytes, burr cells, helmet cells, marked reticulocytosis (with hemolytic anemia), and elevated creatinine and BUN are typical. Fibrin split products occasionally elevated but usually normal. Negative Coombs test and normal PT and PTT are typical

- •BONE MARROW ASPIRATION AND BIOPSY - Normal or elevated megakaryocytes may be seen.

von HIPPEL-LINDAU DISEASE
- •BLOOD - Occasionally elevated VMA, catecholamines and metanephrines if associated with a pheochromocytoma.
- •RADIOGRAPHY
  CT/MRI - May show cystic changes in the kidneys and pancreas, cerebral neoplasm or cerebellar hemorrhage.
  Angiography - May show brain stem vascular malformations.

HODGKIN'S DISEASE
- •BLOOD - Anemia in advanced disease. Elevated ESR and serum copper are common.
- •BIOPSY - Lymph node: typically shows reactive lymphocytes, plasma cells and malignant Sternberg-Reed cells (not pathognomonic).
- •Studies used in staging the exent of adenopathy include: Chest.
- •Radiograph, CT Scan of chest and abdomen, and lymphangiogram. Bone Marrow aspirate and biopsy to detect presence of malignant cells.

IDIOPATHIC THROMBOCYTOPENIC PURPURA
- •BLOOD - Decreased platelet count. Negative Coombs' test and normal RBC morphology are typical. Platelet bound IgG /IgM is usually increased. PT and PTT is typically normal.
- •BONE MARROW ASPIRATION AND BIOPSY - Megakaryocytic hyperplasia is seen.

LEUKEMIAS
AML
- •BLOOD - Hemoglobin, hematocrit and platelet count are typically decreased. WBC is variable, with increased immature WBC on smear. Uric acid is usually elevated.

•BONE MARROW ASPIRATION AND BIOPSY - Immature WBC's with maturation arrest and increased myeloid/erythroid ratio are seen.
•CYTOGENIC ANALYSIS - Usually abnormal.
•CYTOCHEMISTRY:
  1. Myeloperoxidase stain or Sudan Black stain of bone marrow specimen will identify myeloid cells.
  2. Nonspecific esterase stain of bone marrow specimen using alpha-naphthyl butyrate substrate will identify monocytic cells.

ALL
•See AML above
•CYTOCHEMISTRY - Terminal Deoxynucleotidyl Transferase Assay will identify lymphoblasts.
•IMMUNOPHENOTYPING - Typically aids in disease subtyping.
•CYTOGENIC ANALYSIS - Is usually abnormal.

CML
•BLOOD - Elevated WBC, normal or decreased hemoglobin and hematocrit and elevated platelet count are typical. On smear, immature WBCs and giant platelets are typical. Uric acid is usually elevated and leukocyte alkaline phosphatase decreased.
•BONE MARROW ASPIRATION AND BIOPSY - Myeloid hyperplasia, left shift (without maturation arrest) and increased myeloid/erythroid ratio are typical.
•CYTOGENIC ANALYSIS - Philadelphia chromosome: t (9;22) is typically positive.

CLL
•BLOOD - Increased WBC with lymphocytosis, normal or decreased hemoglobin, hematocrit and platelet count are typically in advanced disease. On smear, lymphocytosis and large number of smudge cells are typical.
•SERUM PROTEIN ELECTROPHORESIS - Hypogammaglobulinemia and occasional monoclonal spike may be seen.
•BONE MARROW ASPIRATION AND BIOPSY - Lymphocytic infiltrate is typical.
•BIOPSY - Lymph node typically shows diffuse effacement by small lymphocytes.

HAIRY CELL LEUKEMIA
•BLOOD - Moderate pancytopenia is typical. On smear: occasionally characteristic hairy cells (cytoplasmic projections) are seen (best

seen with phase microscope, but electron microscopy may be necessary for visualization.)
- BONE MARROW ASPIRATION AND BIOPSY - May show replacement by mononuclear cells and stain is often positive for TRAP (Tartrate Resistant Acid Phosphatase).

METHEMOGLOBINEMIA
CONGENITAL
- BLOOD - Methemoglobin level is typically increased as is a decrease in NADH-methemoglobin reductase.
- Spectrophotometric Analysis of Hemolysate - May identify HbM.
- Hemoglobin Electrophoresis typically identifies HbM.

ACQUIRED
- BLOOD - Increased methemoglobin level and normal level of NADH-methemoglobin reductase are typical.

MULTIPLE MYELOMA
- BLOOD - Hemoglobin and hematocrit are usually decreased. Occasional neutropenia, normal or decreased platelets, rouleaux formation, elevated ESR, elevated uric acid, normal BUN/creatinine and elevated protein on electrophoresis (shows immunoglobulin spike). Quantitative immunoglobulins may show elevation of predominant immunoglobulin with depression of other immunoglobulin types.
- BONE MARROW ASPIRATION AND BIOPSY - Plasma cell infiltrate is typical.
- URINALYSIS - Urine protein dipstick may be negative yet increased Bence-Jones protein may be found with sulfosalicylic acid test or immunoelectrophoresis.
- RADIOGRAPHY - Bone films may show lytic lesions and/or diffuse osteoporosis.

MYELOFIBROSIS (AGNOGENIC MYLEOID METAPLASIA)
- BLOOD - Hemoglobin and hematocrit are usually decreased. On smear: teardrop cells, basophilic stippling, bizarre RBC shapes and giant platelets.are common. May have leukocytosis with left shift and occasionally leukopenia. Later in disease, elevated total bilirubin and increased alkaline phosphatase may be seen.
- BONE MARROW ASPIRATION AND BIOPSY - Fibrosis is typically seen.

NON-HODGKIN'S LYMPHOMA
- BLOOD - Normal to decreased hemoglobin and hematocrit, variable neutrophil and platelet counts, elevated serum LDH and abnormal lymphocytes on smear may be seen. Electrophoresis may show an immunoglobulin spike.
- BONE MARROW ASPIRATION AND BIOPSY - May show lymphocytic infiltrate.
- BIOPSY - Lymph Node: may show lymphocytes in varying degrees of differentiation and varied structural patterns.
- RADIOGRAPHY
  Chest Radiogram or CT - Mediastinal/hilar adenopathy may be present.
  Abdominal or Pelvic CT - Adenopathy may be present.
  Lymphangiogram - May identify subtle filling defects in lymph nodes.

POLYCYTHEMIA VERA
- BLOOD - Elevated hemoglobin and hematocrit. Normal or elevated 51-Cr-labeled red-cell mass and 131-I-Labled albumin. Normal or decreased platelet count, MCV, MCH, and MCHC are typical. Vitamin B_{12}, B_{12} binding capacity, leukocyte alkaline phosphatase, and uric acid may be elevated. On smear: poikilocytosis, anisocytosis, myelocytes, metamyelocytes, and increased basophils are typical.
- BONE MARROW ASPIRATION AND BIOPSY - Hyperplasia of all elements and increased reticulin are typical.

PROSTATE CANCER
- BLOOD - Acid phosphatase may be elevated. Alkaline phosphatase may be elevated if metastases are present.
- RADIOGRAPHY- Skeletal may show lytic or blastic changes. IVP may show obstruction. CT may show the extent of involvement.
- BIOPSY (Needle) - Typically shows adenocarcinoma.

PURE RED CELL APLASIA
- BLOOD - Hemoglobin and hematocrit are typically decreased. Iron levels are typically high during crisis. Iron binding capacity (almost complete saturation during crisis) and high level of erythropoietin are typical. On smear, reticulocytopenia is typical.
- CXR/CT - Thymic enlargement may be present.

•BONE MARROW ASPIRATION AND BIOPSY - Virtual absence of
   nucleated erythroid cells with normal myeloid cells and
   megakaryocytes are characteristic.

THALASSEMIAS

Beta (Major)
•BLOOD - Hemoglobin and hematocrit are usually decreased.
   Smear: hypochromic microcytic target cells, elevated reticulocyte
   count, extreme poikilocytosis with inclusion bodies (when
   incubated with methyl violet) are typical. Iron and ferritin may be
   normal or high depending on the treatment status of the patient
   (ie. transfusions).
•HEMOGLOBIN ELECTROPHORESIS - If Beta (0) = HbA is absent
   then HbF 98%, and HbA_2=2%, if Beta (+) =HbA is present HbF =
   60-95%.

Beta (Minor)
•BLOOD - Elevated red cell count (often > 5,000,000/cc^3) and
   decreased hemoglobin, hematocrit and MCV are typical. Ferritin
   is usually normal.
•HEMOGLOBIN ELECTROPHORESIS - Elevated HbA_2 and HbF are
   typical.

Alpha
Alpha (Hydrops Fetalis - complete absence of alpha chains)
   (incompatible with life).
Alpha (= H Disease, absence of 3 of 4 Alpha genes)
   •BLOOD - On smear: hypochromic, microcytic anemia, target cells
      and anisopoikilocytosis with elevated reticulocytes are typical.
   •HEMOGLOBIN ELECTROPHORESIS - HbH: 4-30% and trace Hb
      (B4) are typical.
   •Hemoglobin H Preparation: Multiple small blue RBC inclusions
      with brilliant cresyl blue preparation is characteristic.
Alpha (Alpha Thalassemia Trait absence of 2 of the 4 genes)
   •BLOOD - On smear: microcytic, hypochromic (mild) anemia with
      normal iron and ferritin levels are typical.
   •HEMOGLOBIN ELECTROPHORESIS - Is typically normal.
   •Simple confirmatory tests not avalilable, usually diagnosed by
      exclusion of other causes of microcytic/hypochromic anemia.
Alpha - Silent carrier state (1 of 4 alpha genes absent).

THROMBOTIC THROMBOCYTOPENIC PURPURA
- •URINE - Proteinuria and micro or gross hematuria are typical.
- •BLOOD - Decreased platelet count, schistocytes, burr cells, helmet cells, marked reticulocytosis (with hemolytic anemia), elevated fibrin split products, negative Coombs test elevated creatinine and LDH, PT and normal PTT may be seen.
- •BIOPSY (Petechiae) - platelet aggregates, small vessel occlusion and endothelial proliferation are typical.
- •BONE MARROW ASPIRATION AND BIOPSY - Normal or elevated megakaryocyte number may be seen.

WALDENSTROMS MACROGLOBULINEMIA
- •BLOOD - Normocytic normochromic anemia is typical. On smear rouleaux formation is common. A monoclonal spike may be seen on serum electrophoresis and on immunoelectrophoresis a monoclonal IgM spike. Serum viscosity may be elevated.
- •BONE MARROW AND ASPIRATION - Infiltration by plasmacytoid lymphocytes is typical.
- •URINE ELECTROPHORESIS - May have Bence-Jones protein.

HEMATOLOGY AND ONCOLOGY REFERENCES

ANEMIAS

1. Finch, C. A., Huebers, H.: Perspectives in iron metabolism. *N. E. J. M.* 1982; 306:1520-1527.
2. Lindenbaum, J.: Status of laboratory testing in the diagnosis of megaloblastic anemia. *Blood* 1983; 61:624-626.
3. Camitta, B. M., Strob, R., Thomas, E. D.: Aplastic anemia. Pathogenesis, diagnosis, treatment and prognosis. *N. E. J. M.* 1982; 306:645-652, 712-718.
4. Swisher, S.N. (ed).: Immune hemolytic anemias. *Semin. Hematol.* 1976; 13:251-253.
5. Palek, J., Samuel, L.: Red cell membrane skeletal defects in hereditary and acquired hemolytic anemias. *Semin. Hematol.* 1983; 20:189-224.
6. Buetler,E.: The sickle cell diseases and related disorders. In Williams, W. J., Beutler, E., Erslev, A. J., Lictman, M. A. (eds), Hematology. Philadelphia, McGraw-Hill. 1983, pp 583-609.
7. Nienhuis, A. W., moderator: Thalassemia major: molecular and clinical aspects. *Ann. Intern. Med.* 1979; 91:883-897.
8. Hansen, R. M., Hanson, G., Anderson, T.: Failure to suspect and diagnose thalassemic syndrome. Interpretation of RBC indices by the nonhematologist. *Arch. Intern. Med.* 1985;145:93-94.

BLADDER CANCER

1. Zingg, E. J., Wallace, D. M. A. (eds). Bladder Cancer, Berlin, New York, Tokyo, Springer-Verlag. 1985.

BLEEDING DISORDERS

1. Fischbach, D. P., Fogdall, R. P.: Coagulation: The essentials. Baltimore, Williams and Wilkins. 1981, pp 87-115.
2. Jagathambal, K., Grunwald, H. W., Rosner, F.: Evaluation and management of the bleeding patient. *Med. Clin. N. Am.* 1981; 65:133-145.

COLD AGGLUTININ SYNDROME

1. Brouet , J. C., Clauvel, J. P., Danon, F., Klein , M., Seligmann, M.: Biologic and clinical significance of cryoglobulins. *Am. J. Med.* 1974; 57:775-788.
2. Pruzanski, W., Shumak, K. H.: Biologic activity of cold-reacting autoantibodies. *N. E. J. M.* 1977; 297:538-542, 583-589.

DISSEMINATED INTRAVASCULAR COAGULATION

1. Fischbach, D. P., Fogdall, R. P. Coagulation. The essentials. Baltimore,Williams and Wilkins. 1981, pp 116-132.
2. Marder, V. J. Consumptive thrombohemorrhagic disorders. In Williams, W. J., Beulter, E., Erslev, A. J., Lictman, M. A. (eds), Hematology. Philadelphia, McGraw-Hill. 1983, pp 1433-1461.

ESSENTIAL THROMBOCYTOSIS

1. Jabaily, J., Iland, H. J., Lazlo, J., et al.: Neurologic manifestations of essential thrombocythemia. *Ann. Intern. Med.* 1983; 99:513-518.
2. Baumann, M. A., Pacheco, J.: Myleoproliferative disorders. In Barnes, H. V. (ed), Clinical Medicine: Selected problems with pathophysiologic correlations. Chicago, Medical Yearbook Publishers. 1988, pp 445-450.

EVAN'S SYNDROME

1. Packman C. H., Leddy J. P. Acquired hemolytic anemia due to warm-reacting autoantibodies. In Williams, W. J., Beulter, E., Erslev, A. J., Lictman, M. A. (eds), Hematology. Philadelphia, McGraw-Hill. 1983, pp 632-641.

GLUCOSE-6-PHOSPHATE DEHYDROGENASE (G-6-PD) DEFICIENCY

1. Valentine, W. M., moderator.: Hemolytic anemias and erythrocyte enzymopathies. *Ann. Intern. Med.* 1985; 103:245-257.

HEMOCHROMATOSIS

1. Finch, C. A., Huebers, H.: Perspectives in iron metabolism. N. E. J. M. 1982; 306:1520-1527.
2. Milder, M. S., Cook, J. D., Stray, S., Finch, C. A.: Idiopathic hemochromatosis: An interim report. *Medicine* 1980; 59:34.

HEMOLYTIC UREMIC SYNDROME

1. Aster, R. H.: Thrombocytopenia due to enhanced platelet destruction. In Williams, W. J., Beutler, E., Erslev, A. J., Lictman,M. A (eds), Hematology. Philadelphia, McGraw-Hill. 1983, pp 1298-1338.

HEREDITARY ELLIPTOCYTOSIS

1. Palek, J., Samuel, L.: Red cell membrane skeletal defects in hereditary and acquired hemolytic anemias. *Semin. Hematol.* 1983; 20:189-224.

HEREDITARY SPHEROCYTOSIS

1. Palek, J., Samuel, L.: Red cell membrane skeletal defects in hereditary and acquired hemolytic anemias. *Semin. Hematol.* 1983; 20:189-224.

HODGKIN'S DISEASE

1. DeVita, V. T., Jaffe, E. S., Helman, S.: Hodgkin's disease and the non-Hodgkin's lymphomas. In DeVita, V. T., Hellman, S., Rosenberg,S. A. (eds). Cancer: Priniciples and practice of oncology, 2nd Ed. Philadelphia, J. P. Lippincott. 1985, pp 1623-1709.

IDIOPATHIC THROMBOCYTOPENIC PURPURA

1. McMillian, R.: Chronic idiopathic thrombocytopenic purpura. *N. E. J. M.* 1981; 304:1135-1146.

LEUKEMIAS

1. Baumann, M. A., Pacheco, J.: Acute non-lymphocytic leukemia. In Barnes, H. V. (ed), Clinical Medicine: Selected Problems with pathophysiologic correlations. Chicago, Medical Yearbook Publishers. 1988, pp 450-455.
2. Jacobs, A. D., Gale, R. P.: Recent advances in the biology and treatment of acute lymphoblastic leukemia in adults. *N. E. J. M.* 1984; 311:1219-1231.
3. Gale, R. P., Foon, K. A.: Chronic lymphocytic leukemia: recent advances in biology and treatment. *Ann. Intern. Med.* 1985; 103:101-119.
4. Koeffler, H. P., Golde, D. W.: Chronic myelogenous leukemia. New Concepts. *N. E. J. M.* 1981; 304:1201-1208, 1269-1274.

METHEMOGLOBULIN

1. Beutler, E.: Methemoglobinemia and sulfhemoglobinemia. In Williams, W. J., Beulter, E., Erslev, A. J., Lictman, M. A. (eds), Hematology. Philadelphia, McGraw-Hill. 1983, pp 604-706.

MULTIPLE MYELOMA

1. McIntrye, O. R.: Current concepts in cancer. Multiple myeloma. *N. E. J. M.* 1979; 301:193-196.
2. Bergsagel, D. E., Rider, W. D.: Plasma cell neoplasms. In Cancer: Principles and Practice of Oncology. DeVita, V. T., Hellman, S., Rosenberg, S. A. (eds), J. P. Lippincott, Philadelphia, 1985, pp 1753-1795.

MULTIPLE ENDOCRINE NEOPLASIAS

1. Brennan, M. F., Macdonald, J. S.: Cancer of the endocrine system. In DeVita, V. T., Hellman, S., Rosenberg, S. (eds), Cancer: Principles and Practice of Oncology, 2nd Ed. New York, J. P. Lippincott. 1985, pp 1179-1241.

MYELOFIBROSIS

1. Varki, A., Lottenberg, R., Griffith, R., Reinhard, E.: The syndrome of idiopathic myelofibrosis. A clinicopathologic review with emphasis on the prognostic variables predicting survival. *Medicine.* 1983; 62:353-371.

2. Baumann, M. A., Pacheco, J.: Myeloproliferative disorders. In Barnes, H. V. (ed), Clinical Medicine: Selected Problems with pathophysiologic correlations. Chicago, Medical Yearbook Publishers. 1988, pp 445-450.

NON-HODGKIN'S LYMPHOMA

1. Hait, W. M., Farber, L., Cadman, E.: Non-hodgkin's lymphoma for the nononcologist. *J. A. M. A.* 1985; 253:1431-1435.

2. Baumann, M. A., Pacheco, J.: Non-hodgkin's lymphoma. In Barnes, H. V. (ed), Clinical Medicine: Selected Problems with patho-physiologic correlations. Chicago, Medical Yearbook   Publishers. 1988, pp 461-466.

PAROXYSMAL NOCTURNAL HEMOGLOBINURIA

1. Rosse, W. F.: Treatment of paroxysmal nocturnal hemoglobinuria. *Blood.* 1982; 60:20-22.

POLYCYTHEMIA VERA

1. Golde, D. W., moderator: Polycythemia: Mechanisms and management. *Ann. Intern. Med.* 1981; 95:71-87.

2. Baumann, M. A., Pacheco, J.: Myeloproliferative disorders. In Barnes, H. V. (ed), Clinical Medicine: Selected Problems with pathophysiologic correlations. Chicago, Medical Yearbook Publishers. 1988, pp 445-450.

PURE RED CELL APLASIA

1. Erslev, A. J.: Pure red cell aplasia. In Williams, W. J., Beulter, E., Erslev, A. J., Lictman, M. A. (eds), Hematology. Philadelphia, McGraw-Hill. 1983, pp 409-417.

SICKLE CELL ANEMIAS

1. Buetler, E.: The sickle cell diseases and related disorders. In Williams, W. J., Buetler, E., Erslev, A. J., Lictman, M. A. (eds), Hematology. Philadelphia, McGraw-Hill. 1983, pp 583-609.

THALASSEMIAS

1. Nienhuis, A. W., moderator: Thalassemia major: molecular and clinical aspects. *Ann. Intern. Med.* 1979; 91:883-897.
2. Hansen, R. M., Hanson, G., Anderson, T.: Failure to suspect and diagnose thalassemic syndrome. Interpretation of RBC indices by the nonhematologist. *Arch. Intern. Med.* 1985; 145:93-94.

THROMBOTIC THROMBOCYTOPENIC PURPURA

1. Crain, S. M., Choudhury, A. M.: Thrombotic thrombocytopenic purpura. A reappraisal. *J. A. M. A.* 1981; 246:1243-1246.
2. Meyes, T. J., Wakem, C. J., Ball, E. D., Tremont, S. J.: Thrombotic thrombocytopenic purpura: combined treatment with plasmapheresis and antiplatelet agents. *Ann. Intern. Med.* 1980; 92:149-155.

WALDENSTROM'S MACROGLOBINEMEIA

1. Kyle, R. A., Garton, J. P.: The spectrum of IgM monoclonal gammopathy in 430 cases. *Mayo. Clin. Proc.* 1987; 62:719-731.

INFECTIOUS DISEASE

The number, types and priority of tests ordered must be individualized for each patient, consequently the tests listed for each disease in this chapter are not prioritized and are not exhaustive.

ABSCESS
GENERAL
- BLOOD - Blood cultures may be positive. WBC and ESR may be elevated.
- NUCLEAR MEDICINE (*ie,* Gallium, Indium or Tc Tagged Leukocyte Scan) - May aid in abscess location and evaluation of size.
- CT SCAN - May aid in abscess location and evaluation of size.
- NEEDLE ASPIRATION - Gram stain and culture may demonstrate organism involved.

ABDOMEN/PELVIS
- BLOOD - WBC and blood cultures may be abnormal.
- CT SCAN - Fluid collection with or without capsule (I.V. contrast may be helpful in identifying abscesses in solid organs), extraluminal gas collection may also be present.
- NUCLEAR SCAN (*ie.* Gallium, Indium or Tc Tagged Leukocyte Scan) - May show involved area.

BRAIN/EPIDURAL
- BLOOD - WBC and blood cultures may be abnormal.
- CT WITH CONTRAST, MRI or NUCLEAR SCAN (*ie.* Gallium, Indium or Tc Tagged Leukocyte Scan) - May show involved area.

ISCHIORECTAL/PSOAS
- BLOOD - WBC and blood cultures may be abnormal.
- RADIOGRAPH / CT SCAN - Fluid collection with or without capsule (I.V. contrast may be helpful in identifying abscesses in solid organs), extraluminal gas collection may also be present.
- NUCLEAR SCAN (*ie.* Gallium, Indium or Tc Tagged Leukocyte Scan) - May show involved area.

LUNG
- SPUTUM - Mixed Gram negative and Gram positive flora (culture or gram stain) may be seen.
- BLOOD - WBC and blood cultures may be abnormal.
- CHEST RADIOGRAPH - Mass with possible air fluid level may be seen.

ASCARIASIS
- STOOL - Parasites may be seen.
- IV Cholangiogram - May show worm within biliary tree.

•CXR - Migratory pulmonary infiltrate may be seen.
•BLOOD - Eosinophilia during larval migration is typical.
•SPUTUM - Larvae and eosinophils may be seen.

CHICKENPOX (VARICELLA-ZOSTER)
•BLOOD - WBC normal or increased, may have increased atypical
  lymphocytes and/or basophils.
•TZANCK SMEARS (with scraping of base of lesion) - May
  demonstrate large epithelial giant cells with intranuclear
  inclusions.

CYTOMEGALOVIRUS
**(pneumonitis, hepatitis, heterophile negative mononucleosis,
esophogitis, enteritis and infrequent neurologic infection)**
•URINE - Large cells with intranuclear inclusions may be seen.
•CULTURE - Virus may be cultured from urine, blood, upper
  respiratory and biopsy material.
•BLOOD - Four fold rise in Anti-CMV antibody. IgM indicates recent
  infection. IgG and IgM may or may not be present in immuno-
  compromised patients.

CONDYLOMA ACUMINATUM
•INSPECTION - May see actual wart. Colposcope often required to
  visualize lesion.
•PAP SMEAR - May be abnormal.

DIARRHEA
•STOOL - Fecal leukocytes may be present in: *Salmonella, Shigella,*
  invasive *E. Coli,* Gonoccocci, *Yersinia, Champylobacter, Vibrio
  Parahemolyticus* and *Clostridium difficile.*
  -ova and parasites found in: *Entamoeba histolytica, Giardia,
  Ascaris strongyloides* and *Cryptosporidium* (seen on acid fast
  stain).
  - STOOL CULTURE: *Salmonella, Shigella, Yersinia,
  Campylobacter* may be identified. Selected stool cultures are
  available for specific organisms - *ie, Vibrio parahemolyticus* and
  Clostridium difficile.

<u>CHRONIC</u> (See Gastroenterology, Diarrhea, chronic)

EPSTEIN-BARR VIRUS INFECTION (EBV)
ACUTE
- •BLOOD - Monospot or heterophile antibody may be positive.
  Lymphocytosis with atypical lymphocytes and elevated IgM EBV
  capsid antibody may be seen.

CONVALESCENT
- •BLOOD - Elevated IgG EBV capsid antibody. Negative IgM E-B Virus
  capsid antibody. Elevated EBV nuclear antigen antibody,
  elevated EBV early antigen antibody, positive Anti-D and negative
  Anti-R are typical.

FILARIASIS (*Wuchenia bancrofti*)
- •LYMPHANGIOGRAPHY - Dilated afferent and small efferent lymph
  vessels may be seen.
- •BIOPSY- Lymph Node: may show organism.
- •BLOOD - Giemsa stain may demonstrate organism and eosinophils.
  Filarial antigens may be detected by complement fixation. IgE and
  ESR are typically increased.
- •URINE - Filarial antigens may be found, with occasional chyluria
  seen.

GONORRHEA
- •GRAM STAIN - Smear from involved site may show intracellular
  Gram negative diplococci.
- •CULTURE - Of involved site on Thayer-Martin media often positive.
- •FLUORESCENT ANTIBODY - Often positive.
- •GONOCOCCAL COMPLEMENT FIXATION TEST - May be positive.

HIV INFECTION
- •BLOOD - Lymphopenia may be present. Anemia, hypergammaglobulinemia and thrombocytopenia are typically seen with
  progressive disease. ELISA and confirmatory Western blot are
  positive. May have T_4 lymphocytes < 400/mm^3, T_8 normal or
  elevated and T_4/T_8 ratio often < 1.0.
- •SKIN TESTS - Anergy often present as disease progresses.
- •RADIOGRAPHY - CXR may show pulmonary infiltrates.
- •BIOPSY - Lymph Node: shows benign lymphoid hyperplasia with
  decreased T_4/T_8 ratio (late in the disease lymphoid depletion may
  be seen). Skin Lesion: may show Kaposi's sarcoma.

•LUMBAR PUNCTURE- CSF: early findings may be consistent with aseptic meningitis, late findings may be characteristic of opportunistic infection or tumor.

KAWASAKI DISEASE (MUCOCUTANEOUS LYMPH NODE SYNDROME)
•See under Rheumatologic diseases.

LEPROSY
•BLOOD - Hypergammaglobulinemia and decreased A/G ratio are typical. If bacteremic, organisms be seen in buffy coat.
  -Acid-fast bacilli may be visualized with Fite-Faraco stain.
•BLOOD CULTURE - Thermolabile, slow-growing organisms are typical.
•BIOPSY
  - Skin: required to make diagnosis:
  -Tuberculoid: Helper T lymphocytes, well-formed granulomas, few organisms are seen.
  -Lepromatous: Suppressor T lymphocytes, numerous bacilli, foam cells, devoid of granulomas are seen.

LEPTOSPIROSIS
•URINE - May find albuminuria, pyuria, cylindruria, proteinuria and positive darkfield examination.
•ECG - Bradycardia; low voltage; nonspecific ST-T wave changes may be seen.
•BLOOD - Elevated WBC and ESR, anemia (in severe disease). May see elevated potassium and BUN. IgM antibodies and elevated direct bilirubin may be seen.
•MACROSCOPIC SLIDE AGGLUTINATION TEST - Positive.
•MICROSCOPIC AGGLUTINATION TEST - Titer ≥1:100, when titer shows a four fold rise from acute to convalescent a more definitive diagnosis is possible (especially when the organism, *Ixodes dammini*, has been isolated).
•CULTURE (EMJH media)
  -First 1-2 weeks: blood or CSF provides the highest positivity.
  -After 1-2 weeks of illness urine provides highest positivity.
•LUMBAR PUNCTURE - CSF: WBC usually < 500/mm^3 with predominantly neutrophils and normal glucose.
•DARK-FIELD EXAM - Of CSF may or may not show organisms.

LYME DISEASE
- •BLOOD - *B. burgdorferi* antibodies (IgM early, IgG late) and total IgM typically elevated. Culture occasionally positive. Serum AST and ESR may be elevated.
- •BIOPSY - Of atypical erythema chronicum migrans: direct immunofluorescence may be positive, spirochetes may be visible in periphery of primary and disseminated erythema chronicum migrans, by Warthin-Starry silver stain.
- •SYNOVIAL FLUID - Elevated WBC mostly neutrophils, culture occasionally positive.

MALARIA
- •BLOOD - WBC decreased or normal, thrombocytopenia, ESR typically very high (>100), thick smear for screening (Giemsa stain), thin smear for identification. Decreased haptoglobin may be seen in blackwater fever. Increased indirect bilirubin and free hemoglobin in the serum, and hemoglobinuria may also be seen.

MENINGITIS
- •BLOOD - WBC and ESR typically elevated in acute bacterial meningitis, blood cultures are usually positive in acute bacterial meningitis.
- •LUMBAR PUNCTURE
  - -CSF pressure may be elevated in: bacterial, fungal and tuberculous meningitis.
  - -CSF WBC is typically elevated, predominantly neutrophils in acute bacterial meningitis, mildly elevated and predominantly mononuclear in viral, fungal and tuberculous meningitis.
  - -CSF protein is typically increased in bacterial including tuberculous meningitis in which levels often exceed 500 mg/dl CSF glucose is typically decreased in bacterial, and moderately decreased in tuberculous and fungal meningitis (usually normal in viral).
  - -CSF Gram stain: may be positive for the organism in acute bacterial.
  - -CSF routine cultures: usually positive in acute bacterial.
  - -CSF AFB smear occasionally positive in tuberculous. meningitis.
  - -CSF AFB culture: usually positive in tuberculous meningitis.

-CSF latex agglutination is occasionally positive for
  Pneumococcal, meningiococcal, Hemophilis influenza type b,
  and Cryptococcal meningitis Cryptococcal Ag (this test allows
  for rapid results) may be positive.
-CSF India Ink preparation is occasionally positive in
  Cryptococcal meningitis.
-CSF fungal cultures are usually positive in fungal meningitis.
-CSF Complement-fixing antibody usually positive in coccidioidal
  meningitis.
-CSF VDRL is usually positive in meningovascular syphilis.
•GRAM STAIN AND CULTURE OF SKIN LESIONS - May show the
  organism in meningococcal and cryptococcal meningitis.

MONONUCLEOSIS
•See Epstein-Barr virus infection.

MUMPS
•BLOOD - Mild leukopenia with relative lymphocytosis (if mumps
  orchitis marked leukocytosis with left shift), increased amylase
  (with salivary adenitis and pancreatis), increased lipase (with
  pancreatitis) may be seen.
•URINE -Transient hematuria may be seen.
•LUMBAR PUNCTURE - CSF: lymphocytic pleocytosis with
  meningitis.
•Antibody Titer, Convalescent - Typically elevated.

OSTEOMYELITIS
•BLOOD - Elevated WBC and ESR may be seen, blood cultures may
  be positive in acute osteomyelitis (especially in children).
•RADIOGRAPHY - May be normal in the first two weeks of illness,
  later signs may include periosteal elevation or erosion followed
  by evidence of increased bone formation (sclerosis) and
  sequestrum or involucrum.
•NUCLEAR SCAN - Technetium or Gallium scans usually show
  uptake in involved area early in the disease process.
•BIOPSY - Bone (needle or open) - for cultural identification of
  bacteria or fungi.

PHARYNGITIS
STREPTOCOCCAL
• Throat Culture - ß-hemolytic *Streptococcus* may be seen.
• Rapid Antigen Detection - (*ie.* latex agglutination). May be positive.

RICKETTSIA
ROCKY MOUNTAIN SPOTTED FEVER (RMSF)
• BLOOD - Thrombocytopenia, occasionally DIC may be seen. Weil-Felix typically positive for OX_{19} and/or OX_2 RMSF complement fixation test: positive if four-fold rise from acute to convalescent serum.
• FLUORESCENT STAINING OF TISSUE SPECIMEN - shows fluorescence of endothelium.
• LUMBAR PUNCTURE - CSF: when meningoencephalitis is suspected, may show slight increase in protein, normal glucose and mild WBC elevation with differential.

RICKETTSIAL POX
• BLOOD - Complement fixation test shows four-fold rise from acute to convalescent (negative Weil-Felix).

Q FEVER
• DIRECT MICROSCOPIC DEMONSTRATION of organism in endothelial cells of skin biopsy.
• RICKETTSIAL ANTIGEN - May be positive in the urine during acute phase.
• BLOOD - Complement fixation test typically shows fourfold rise from acute to convalescent (negative Weil-Felix).

SEPSIS (BACTERIAL)
• BLOOD
    -WBC usually 15,000-30,000, platelets usually decreased, hemoglobin initially increased then decreased as fluid volume replaced, clotting time increases with clotting factor depletion, hyponatremia, hypochloremia, decreased bicarbonate and increased lactate may be seen.
    -ABG: early: usually pCO_2 decreased and pH increased. Late: pCO_2 is variable.
    -Electrolytes: elevated BUN and creatinine may be seen.
    -Gram stain of buffy coat may be positive in sepsis
      (*ie.* pneumococcal and meningococcal).

134

-Latex agglutination may be helpful (*ie.* pneumococcal,
   meningococcal staphylococcal or fungal).
•BLOOD CULTURES - are typically positive.
•URINE - Creatinine may be increased.

TOXOPLASMOSIS
•BLOOD - Normal WBC with slight lymphocytosis or monocytosis may
   be seen. Liver function tests may be elevated. Sabin-Feldman
   dye test, IgG-indirect fluorescent antibody test may be positive.

TUBERCULOSIS
•BLOOD - Peripheral blood may show monocytosis.
•CHEST RADIOGRAPH - Variable possibilities include: multinodular
   infiltrates in apical posterior segments of upper lobes, Ghon
   complex, miliary pattern or cavitary disease (in extrapulmonary
   Tuberculosis CXR may be negative).
•Tubercle Bacilli - May be seen in sputum, urine, body fluids or tissue
   (caseating granuloma with Langerhans giant cells).

URINARY TRACT INFECTIONS
•URINE - Gram stain of uncentrifuged urine may correlate with the
   number of organisms (*ie.* when > 1-2 bacteria /oil emersion
   field may correspond to 100,000 organisms/ml).
-Gram stain of sediment may reveal the pseudohyphal elements
   of yeast (may correlate with tissue invasion of bladder or
   upper tract).
-Elevated WBC, RBCs and casts may be seen.
-Fluorescent antibody coating of bacteria may correlate with
   upper urinary tract infection in females and may be falsely
   positive in men with prostatitis.

INFECTIOUS DISEASE REFERENCES

ABSCESS
1. In Sabiston (ed): Textbook of surgery, 13th Ed. Philadelpha, W.B. Saunders. 1986.

ASCARIASIS
1. Mahmoud, A.A.F. Intestinal Nematodes (Roundworms). In Mandell, G.L., Douglas, R.G., Jr, Bennett , J.E. (eds): Principles and Practice of Infectious Disease, 2nd Ed. New York, John Wiley and Sons. 1985, pp 1565-1566.

CHICKENPOX
1. Brunell, P.A. Varicella-Zoster Virus. In Mandell, G.L., Douglas, R.G., Jr., Bennett, J.E (eds): Principles and Practice of Infectious Disease, 2nd Ed. New York, John Wiley and Sons. 1985, pp 952-959.

CONDYLOMA LATA
1. Rein, M.F. Skin and mucous membrane lesions. In Mandell, G.L., Douglas, R.G., Jr., Bennett, J.E. (eds): Principles and Practice of Infectious Disease, 2nd Ed. New York, John Wiley and Sons. 1985, p 714.

CYTOMEGALOVIRUS (CMV)
1. Ho, M. Cytomegalovirus. In Mandell, G.L., Douglas, R.G., Jr., Bennett, J.E. (eds): Principles and Practice of Infectious Disease, 2nd Ed. New York, John Wiley and Sons. 1985, pp 960-969.

EPSTEIN-BARR VIRUS (EBV)
1. Schooley, R.T., Dolin, R. Epstein-Barr virus (Infectious Mono-nucleosis). In Mandell, G.L., Douglas, R.G., Jr., Bennett, J.E. (eds): Principles and Practice of Infectious Disease, 2nd Ed. New York, John Wiley and Sons. 1985, pp 971-979.

FILARIASIS
1. Orihel, T.C., Ash, L.R: Tissue Helminthes. In Lennette, E.H., Balows, A., Hausler, W.J., Jr., Shadomy, H.J. (eds): Manual of Clinical Microbiology, 4th Ed. Washington, American Society for Micro-biology. 1985, pp 651-659.

2. Ottesen, E.A.: Filariasis and tropical eosinophilia. In Warren, K.S., Mahmond, A.A.F. (eds): Tropical and Geographical Medicine. New York, McGraw Hill Book Co. 1984, pp 390-412.
3. Smith, J.W.: Medical parasitology in the United States: approach to laboratory diagnosis. In Lorian, V (ed): Significance of Medical Microbiology in the Care of Patients, 2nd Ed. Baltimore, Williams and Wilkins 1982, pp 197-238.

GONORRHEA

1. Ward, T.T., Szeberyi, S.E.: Sexually transmitted diseases. In Reese, R.E., Douglas, R.G. Jr. (eds): A Practical Approach to Infectious Diseases, 2nd Ed. Boston, Little, Brown and Co. 1986, pp 359-384.
2. Black, J.R., Sparling, P.F.: Neisseria gonorrhoeae. In Mandell, G.L., Douglas, RG, Jr, Bennett, JE (eds): Principles and Practice of Infectious Disease, 2nd Ed. New York, John Wiley and Sons. 1985, pp 1195-1205.
3. Morrello, J.A., Janda, W.M., Bornhoff: Neisseria and branhamella. In Lennette, E.H., Balows, A., Hausler, W.J., Jr., Shadomy, H.J. (eds): Manual of Clinical Microbiology, 4th Ed. Washington, American Society for Microbiology. 1985, pp 176-192.

HUMAN IMMUNODEFICIENCY VIRUS (AIDS)

1. Masur, H., Macher, A.M.. Acquired Immune Deficiency Syndrome (AIDS). In Mandell, GL, Douglas, RG Jr, Bennett , JE (eds): Principles and Practice of Infectious Disease, 2nd Ed. New York, John Wiley and Sons. 1985, pp 1670-73.
2. Carlson, J.R., Bryant, M.L., Hinrichs, S.H., et al: AIDS serology testing in low- and high-risk groups, JAMA, 1985; 253(23): 3405-3408.
3. Weiss, S.H., Goedert, J.J., Sarngadharan, M.G.: Screening test for T+HTLV-III (AIDS agent) antibodies, JAMA, 1985; 253(2): 221-225.
4. Abramowicz, M., ed: Screening for AIDS, The Medical Letter, 1985; 27: 29-30.
5. Sivak, S.L., Wormser, G.P.: Predictive value of a screening test for antibodies to HTLV-III, Am. J. of Clin. Path. 1986; 85(6): 700-703.
6. Barnes, D.M.: New questions about AIDS test accuracy, Science, 1987; 238:884-885.

LEPROSY

1. Bullock, W.E.. *Mycobacterium Leprae*. In Mandell, G.L., Douglas, R.G., Jr., Bennett, J.E. (eds): Principles and Practice of Infectious Disease, 2nd Ed. New York, John Wiley and Sons. 1985, pp 1407-1409.

LEPTOSPIROSIS

1. Alexander, A.D. Leptospira. In Lennette, E.H., Balows, A., Hausler, W.J. Jr., Shadomy, H.J. (eds): Manual of Clinical Microbiology, 4th Ed. Washington, American Society for Microbiology. 1985, pp 473-478.
2. Farrar, W.E. Leptospira species (leptospirosis). In Mandell, G.L., Douglas, R.G., Jr., Bennett , J.E (eds): Principles and Practice of Infectious Disease, 2nd Ed. New York, John Wiley and Sons. 1985, pp 1338-1341.
3. Johnson, R.C. Leptospirosis. In Warren, K.S., Mahmond, A.A.F. (eds): Tropical and Geographical Medicine. New York, McGraw Hill Book Co. 1984, pp 839-843.

LYME DISEASE

1. Steere, A.C., Malawista, S.E. Lyme Disease. In Mandell, G.L., Douglas, R.G., Jr, Bennett , J.E. (eds): Principles and Practice of Infectious Disease, 2nd Ed. New York, John Wiley and Sons. 1985, pp 1343-1348.

MALARIA

1. Wyler, D.J. *Plasmodium* species. In Mandell, G.L., Douglas, R.G.,Jr., Bennett , JE (eds): Principles and Practice of Infectious Disease, 2nd Ed. New York, John Wiley and Sons. 1985, pp 1514-1522.

MENINGITIS

1. Washington, J. A. Bacteria, Fungi, and Parasites. In Mandell, G.L., Douglas, R.G., Jr., Bennett , J.E. (eds): Principles and Practice of Infectious Disease, 2nd Ed. New York, John Wiley and Sons. 1985, pp 118-120.

MUMPS

1. Norrby, E. Mumps Virus. In Lennette, E.H., Balows, A., Hausler, W.J., Jr., Shadomy, H.J. (eds): Manual of Clinical Microbiology, 4th Ed. Washington, American Society for Microbiology. 1985, pp 774-778.
2. Baum, S.G., Litman, N. Mumps Virus. In Mandell, G.L., Douglas, R.G., Jr., Bennett , J.E. (eds): Principles and Practice of Infectious Disease, 2nd Ed. New York, John Wiley and Sons. 1985, pp 871-876.
3. Toplin, M.D., Schauf, V. Mumps virus. In Belshe, R.B. (ed): Textbook of Human Virology. Littleton, P.S.G Publishing Co. 1984, pp 311-331.

OSTEOMYELITIS

1. Norden, C.W. Osteomyelitis. In Mandell, G.L., Douglas, R.G., Jr, Bennett , J.E. (eds): Principles and Practice of Infectious Disease, 2nd Ed. New York, John Wiley and Sons. 1985, pp 704-711.

PHARYNGITIS

1. Gwaltney, J.M. Pharyngitis. In Mandell, G.L., Douglas, R.G., Jr., Bennett , J.E. (eds): Principles and Practice of Infectious Disease, 2nd Ed. New York, John Wiley and Sons. 1985, pp 355-358.

RICKETTSIA

1. Woodward, T.E., Osterman, J.V. Rickettsial Diseases. In Warren, K.S., Mahmond, A.A.F. (eds): Tropical and Geographical Medicine. New York, McGraw Hill Book Co. 1984, pp 873-885.
2. Woodward, W.E., Hornick, R.B. Rickettsia rickettsii (Rocky Mountain Spotted Fever). In Mandell, GL, Douglas, R.G., Jr, Bennett , J.E (eds): Principles and Practice of Infectious Disease, 2nd Ed. New York, John Wiley and Sons. 1985, pp 1082-1087.
3. Saah, A.J., Hornick, R.B. Rickettsia akari (rickettsial pox). In Mandell, G.L., Douglas, R.G., Jr., Bennett , J.E. (eds): Principles and Practice of Infectious Disease, 2nd Ed. New York, John Wiley and Sons. 1985, pp 1087-1088.
4. Saah, A.J., Hornick, R.B. Coxiella burnetii (Q fever). In Mandell, G.L., Douglas, R.G., Jr, Bennett , J.E. (eds): Principles and Practice of Infectious Disease, 2nd Ed. New York, John Wiley and Sons. 1985, pp 1088-1090.

SEPSIS (BACTERIAL)

1. Aronson, M.D., Bor, D.H. Blood cultures. In Sox, H.C., Jr. (ed): Common Diagnostic Tests: Use and Interpretation. Philadelphia, American College of Physicians 1987, pp 176-195.
2. Folyzer, M.A. Reese, R.E. Bacteremias and sepsis. In Reese, R.E., Douglas, R.G., Jr. (eds): A Practical Approach to Infectious Diseases, 2nd Ed. Boston, Little, Brown and Co. 1986, pp 47-74.
3. Dale, D.C, Petersdorf, R.G. Septic shock. In Braunwald, E. (ed): Harrison's Principles of Internal Medicine, 11th Ed. New York, McGraw-Hill Book Co.1987, pp 474-478.

TOXOPLASMOSIS

1. McCabe, R.E., Remington, J.S. *Toxoplasma gondii*. In Mandell, G.L., Douglas, R.G., Jr, Bennett , J.E. (eds): Principles and Practice of Infectious Disease, 2nd Ed. New York, John Wiley and Sons. 1985, pp 1546.

TUBERCULOSIS

1. Phair, JP. Delayed hypersensitivity skin testing: uses and pitfalls. In Remington, JS, Swartz, MN (eds): Current Clinical Topics in Infectious Diseases, vol. 9. New York, McGraw-Hill Book Co. 1988, pp 215-221.
2. Sommers, H Ml Good, R.C. Mycobacterium. In Lennette, E.H., Balows, A., Hausler, W.J., Jr, Shadomy, H.J. (eds): Manual of Clinical Microbiology, 4th Ed. Washington, American Society for Microbiology. 1985, pp 216-248.
3. Des Prez, R.M., Goodwin, R.A., Jr. Mycobacterial diseases. In Mandell, GL, Douglas, RG, Jr, Bennett , JE (eds): Principles and Practice of Infectious Disease, 2nd Ed. New York, John Wiley and Sons. 1985, pp 1383-1406.

URINARY TRACT INFECTIONS

1. Ronald, A.R., Conway, B. An approach to urinary tract infections in ambulatory women. In Remington, J.S., Swartz, M.N. (eds): Current Clinical Topics in Infectious Diseases, vol. 9. New York, McGraw-Hill Book Co. 1988, pp 76-125.
2. Sobel, J.D., Kaye, D. Urinary tract infections. In Mandell, G.L., Douglas, R.G., Jr, Bennett , J.E. (eds): Principles and Practice of Infectious Disease, 2nd Ed. New York, John Wiley and Sons. 1985, pp 426-452.
3. Komaroff, A.L. Urinalysis and urine cultures in women with dysuria. In Sox,H.C., Jr. (ed): Common Diagnostic Tests: Use and Interpretation.
Philadelphia, American College of Physicians. 1987, pp 238-256.

NEPHROLOGY

The number, types and priority of tests ordered must be individualized for each patient, consequently the tests listed for each disease in this chapter are not prioritized and are not exhaustive.

ALLERGIC INTERSTITIAL NEPHRITIS
- URINE - Eosinophils found in giemsa or Wright stained sediment.
- BLOOD - May be elevated eosinophil count.

ACUTE TUBULAR NECROSIS (ATN)
- URINE - Sodium elevated (> 20 meq/L), fractional excretion of Na
  elevated >3%, osmolality low, may be oliguric anuric or polyuric.
  Although urine electrolytes may be diagnostically useful there
  are exceptions *ie.* burns, sepsis, contrast induced ATN, hemo-
  globinuria, myoglobinuria and severe hepatic disease.
  - Microscopic exam non-specific. May have dirty brown granular
    and/or hyaline casts and epithelial cells.
  - Proteinuria and hematuria are not features of ATN.
- BLOOD - Elevated BUN and Creatinine.

ALPORT'S SYNDROME (HEREDITARY NEPHRITIS)
- URINE - Microscopic or gross hematuria, worse with exercise.
  Nephrotic syndrome occurs occasionally, slowly progressive
  renal failure.
- AUDIOMETRY - High frequency sensory neural deafness.
- BLOOD - May show thrombocytopenia (megathrombocytopenia).

AMYLOIDOSIS, RENAL
- URINE - Proteinuria (often more than a gram/day) Light chain may
  or may not be present.
- BLOOD - Hypoalbuminemia may be seen. May have monoclonal
  protein pattern.
- BIOPSY - Abdominal fat pad. Rectal or kidney biopsy may be
  necessary for diagnosis. Typical congo-red positive material is
  diagnostic.

ANALGESIC NEPHROPATHY (see PAPILLARY NECROSIS)

ATHEROEMBOLIC RENAL DISEASE
- BLOOD - BUN, creatinine elevated. Eosinophilia is fairly common.
  ESR may be elevated.
- URINE - May show increased white and red cells. Proteinuria is
  variable.

- •SKIN BIOPSY - Biopsy of affected skin (with livido reticularis or gangrene) may demonstrate cholesterol cleft in subdermal arterial wall.
- •KIDNEY BIOPSY - Presence of cholesterol cleft in glomeruli is diagnostic.

BARTTER'S SYNDROME
- •URINE - Potassium and chloride levels elevated.
- •BLOOD - Hypokalemia, hypomagnesemia, hypochloremic metabolic alkalosis. Renin, aldosterone and uric acid are typically elevated.

BERGER'S DISEASE (IGA-IGG NEPHROPATHY)
- •URINE - Hematuria.
- •KIDNEY BIOPSY - IgA deposits present in the glomeruli.

CALCULI
- •URINE - Microscopic hematuria, 24 hour urine sample may show hypercalciuria (with calcium stones), hyperuricosuria (with calcium or uric acid stones), hyperoxaluria (with Calcium-oxalate stones) and positive nitroprusside test for cystine stones. Positive culture suggests possibility of struvite stone or secondary urinary tract infection. Urine pH may be high in renal tubular acidosis type I.
- •BLOOD - Elevations of calcium, uric acid, and PTH, hyperchloremic acidosis in renal tubular acidosis type I may be seen.
- •RADIOGRAPHY
  - -Flat plate of abdomen may show calculi, serial studies may show movement of calculi.
  - -IVP - May show calculi.

CANCER (KIDNEY)
<u>GENERAL</u>
- •RENAL ULTRASOUND - A simple cyst, solid or complex mass may be seen.
- •I.V.P. - "Mass Effect".
- •CYST ASPIRATION
  - -Simple cyst: Clear fluid, negative cytology.
  - -Complex cyst: May be hemorrhagic and may have malignant cells on cytology.

•CT SCAN - May help differentiate benign cyst from angiomyolipoma
as well as vascular and solid tumors.
•ANGIOGRAM - Neovascularization suggests malignancy.

RENAL CELL CARCINOMA
•URINE - Hematuria typically without proteinuria.
•BLOOD - ESR may be elevated , may have anemia, polycythemia,
hypercalcemia. ACTH-like factor leading to Cushing's syndrome
may occur.
•ARTERIOGRAPHY - Highly vascular mass.
•CT SCAN with contrast - Mass may be visualized.

WILM'S TUMOR
•URINE - microscopic or gross hematuria often with hypertension.
•RENAL ULTRASOUND - Mass seen.
•CT SCAN - Mass seen.

DIABETES INSIPIDUS
NEPHROGENIC DIABETES INSIPIDUS
•URINE - Failure to concentrate urine after 12-18 Hrs. of water
restriction, *ie,* failure to raise urine osmolality above that of
plasma in response to exogenous ADH.
•BLOOD - Normal or increased plasma vasopressin levels,
osmolality elevated.

SIADH (SYNDROME OF INAPPROPRIATE ADH SECRETION)
•URINE - Osmolality inappropriately high when compared to serum
osmolality.
•BLOOD - Decreased osmolality, sodium, uric acid and urea nitrogen.

DIABETIC NEPHROPATHY
•BLOOD - BUN and creatinine may not be elevated early.
•URINE - Proteinuria invariably present. Nephrotic syndrome may be
seen.
•KIDNEY BIOPSY - Shows basement membrane thickening with or
without nodular sclerosis. Typical Kimmelstiel-Wilson changes
present in only 30% of cases.

FABRY'S DISEASE
•BLOOD - Decreased alpha-galactosidase activity.
•URINE - Lipid-laden epithelial cells may be seen. Hematuria and
proteinuria often present.

•KIDNEY BIOPSY - May show increased trihexosylceramide.

FAMILIAL HYPOCALCIURIC HYPOCALCEMIA
•BLOOD - Elevated calcium (PTH normal).
•URINE - Decreased calcium.

FANCONI'S SYNDROME
•URINE - Aminoaciduria, glycosuria, phosphaturia and bicarbonaturia are typical.
•BLOOD - Hypokalemia, low bicarbonate, hypophosphatemia, and hypouricemia may be seen.

GLOMERULONEPHRITIS
GENERAL
•URINE - Hematuria and/or red cell casts, proteinuria (quantitative analysis may be helpful).
•BLOOD - The following tests may be needed for specific diagnosis: Hepatitis B, Surface Ag, C3 and C4, cryoglobulins, ANA, Anti-neutrophil cytoplasmic antibody (ANCA), ASO, Streptozyme, Anti-glomerular basement membrane antibody.
•KIDNEY BIOPSY - May confirm the diagnosis and help distinguish types.

POLYARTERITIS NODOSA
•BLOOD - Anti-neutrophil cytoplasmic antibody (ANCA): Positive only in microscopic Polyarteritis Nodosa.
•RENAL BIOPSY - Necrotizing glomerulonephritis is typical.
•RENAL ANGIOGRAM - Aneurysms of the medium sized arteries may be seen.

POSTSTREPTOCOCCAL GLOMERULONEPHRITIS
•THROAT or SKIN CULTURES - Group A ß-hemolytic Streptococcus may be found.
•BLOOD - ESR and cryoglobulins may be elevated. May show positive ASO, or streptozyme antibody. Decreased C3 and C4 complement levels are typical.
•KIDNEY BIOPSY - Shows diffuse proliferative glomerulonephritis.

WEGNER'S GRANULOMATOSIS
•BLOOD - Elevated BUN and creatinine, anti-neutrophil cytoplasmic antibody (ANCA) may be positive.

-Normochromic anemia may be seen. Mild leukocytosis with
  some patients demonstrating eosinophilia. ESR may be
  elevated and very high.
•URINE - Hematuria and proteinuria.
•RADIOLOGY - CXR may show nodular or cavitary lesions.
•KIDNEY BIOPSY - Focal necrotizing glomerulonephritis.

GOODPASTURE'S SYNDROME
•URINE - Proteinuria with red cells and casts may be seen.
•BLOOD - Antiglomerular basement membrane antibody may be
  present.
•KIDNEY BIOPSY - Linear immunofluorescent deposits, focal or
  diffuse glomerulonephritis.

HEMOLYTIC UREMIC SYNDROME
•BLOOD - Anemia with peripheral smear showing fragmented red
  cells. Platelets often low. BUN and creatinine elevated.
  Fibrinogen and fibrinogen degradation products (FDP) level
  variable. Reticulocyte count elevated. Coombs negative.
•URINE - Proteinuria and hematuria are typical.
•KIDNEY BIOPSY - Microangiopathy indistinguishable from
  Thrombotic Thrombocytopenic Purpura, Progressive Systemic
  Sclerosis and malignant hypertension.

HEPATORENAL SYNDROME
•BLOOD - Elevated BUN and creatinine and liver function tests.
•URINE - Urine Sodium extremely low (<10 meq/L), fractional
  excretion of urinary sodium (FENA) very low (<1%).
  Indistinguishable from prerenal azotemia.

INFARCTON (RENAL)
•URINE - Microscopic or gross hematuria.
•RENAL VASCULAR SCINTIRADIOGRAPHY - Shows focal deficit or
  absent perfusion.

LEAD NEPHROPATHY
•URINE - Mild proteinuria, normal urine sediment, positive EDTA
  24 hour urine lead (>600 µg of lead excreted in 24 hr. sample)
  are typical.
•BLOOD - Elevated serum lead unusual. Azotemia,elevated ESR,
  anemia and sideroblastosis are typical.
•RADIOLOGY - Lead lines (at metaphyseal plate in children).

•KIDNEY BIOPSY - Interstitial nephritis and proximal tubular nuclear inclusion bodies.

LIDDLE'S SYNDROME (PSEUDOHYPERALDOSTRONISM)
•URINE - Hyperkaluria.
•BLOOD - Hypokalemia, hypochloremic metabolic alkalosis (normal or low aldosterone levels help distinguish Liddle's from Bartter's).

MEDULLARY CYSTIC DISEASE
•BLOOD - Elevated BUN and creatinine often present in late stages.
•I.V.P. - Small kidneys, poorly opacified cysts of varying sizes may be seen in the medulla or scattered throughout the kidneys.
•RENAL ULTRASOUND - Widened central echo pattern due to numerous small medullary cysts.

MEDULLARY SPONGE KIDNEY
•URINE - Hematuria.
•RADIOLOGY - Flat plate of Abdomen may show nephrocalcinosis.
•I.V.P. - Radial, linear striations in the papillae, or retained dye in the ectatic collection ducts.

MYELOMA, KIDNEY
•URINE - Bence-Jones protein may be present. Negative urine protein by dipstick and strongly positive by SSA.
•BLOOD - Elevated monoclonal IgG, IgA, or IgM on immuno-electrophoresis. Hypercalcemia, hyperuricemia often present. Anemia usually present.
•RADIOLOGY - Standard bone films may demonstrate punched out lesions.

MYOGLOBINURIA
•URINE - Brown-rust color and elevated myoglobin, strongly positive occult blood test in the absence of significant RBCs on microscopic urine examination.
•BLOOD - Elevated myoglobin may or may not be present, elevated CPK.

NEPHROTIC SYNDROME
•BLOOD - Low albumin, high cholesterol and triglycerides. BUN and creatinine may be normal.

•URINE - 24 hour urine protein exceeds 3 grams.
•KIDNEY BIOPSY - Biopsy may show any primary or secondary
  glomerular disease.

OBSTRUCTIVE UROPATHY
•ULTRASOUND of KIDNEY - Hydronephrosis.
•POST-VOID STRAIGHT CATHETERIZATION OF BLADDER - Often
  greater than 100 cc urine obtained, if obstruction is at the urethral
  level.

ORTHOSTATIC PROTEINURIA
•URINE - Split collection of urine: 12 hours of urine collected from
  patient while ambulatory shows more than 1 gram of protein, and
  12 hours of urine collected while at strict bed rest shows less than
  1 gram of protein.

PAPILLARY NECROSIS
•URINE - Sterile pyuria with tubular epithelial celluria, hematuria,
  proteinuria, WBC, casts, impaired capacity to concentrate urine,
  fragments of necrosed papilla may be seen.
•BLOOD - Anemia, elevated BUN and creatinine.
•I.V.P. or RETROGRADE PYELOGRAPHY - Ring sign, scarred kidney.
• ULTRASOUND/CT SCAN- Calcified papilla.

POLYCYSTIC KIDNEY DISEASE
•URINE - Concentrating ability may be decreased but diluting ability
  is usually not affected. Hematuria and rarely proteinuria may be
  present.
•BLOOD - Elevated hematocrit (secondary to elevated erythropoietin)
  may be present. BUN and Creatinine elevated in late stages.
•RENAL ULTRASOUND- Shows large areas of low echogenicity in
  the kidney.
•CT SCAN- May help differentiate solid from liquid masses.

POSTSTREPTOCOCCAL GLOMERULONEPHRITIS
(SEE GLOMERULONEPHRITIS)

PRE-RENAL AZOTEMIA
•URINE - Urine sodium is low (<20meq/L). Typically urine osmolality
  is high (>500) and fractional excretion of urinary sodium (FENa)
  is low (<1%). There are exceptions (see ATN).

PYELONEPHRITIS, ACUTE
- BLOOD - Elevated WBC.
- URINE - Pyuria with leukocyte casts in urine and hematuria may be seen. Positive urine culture,bacteria on gram stain are typical.

RAPIDLY PROGRESSIVE GLOMERULONEPHRITIS (RPGN)
- BLOOD - Relative rapid rise of BUN and creatinine from normal to very high levels within several days to weeks.
- URINE - Proteinuria and hematuria with or without red cell casts are common.
- KIDNEY BIOPSY - Usually shows crescentric glomerulonephritis (details may vary).

REFLUX NEPHROPATHY (VESICO-URETERAL REFLUX)
- URINE - May show pyuria and bacteruria. Proteinuria may be present in late stages.
- VOIDING CYSTOURETHROGRAM - Reflux of contrast dye into ureter.
- ISOTOPIC CYSTOGRAPH - Shows reflux and is less hazardous than contrast studies.

RENAL ARTERY STENOSIS/RENOVASCULAR HYPERTENSION
- BLOOD - May have hypokalemia. Plasma Renin Activity (PRA) may be elevated (50-60%).
- RAPID SEQUENCE I.V.P. - may show delay in visualization of affected kidney. Affected kidney smaller. Delayed persistent image of affected kidney.
- RADIONUCLEOTIDE RENOGRAM/RENAL SCAN - Delay in rate of rise of tracer and time to peak in the kidney.
- DIGITAL SUBTRACTION ANGIOGRAM (DSA) - May show obstruction.
- SELECTIVE RENAL ANGIOGRAM - May show obstruction.
- RENAL VEIN RENIN RATIO (RVR) - A lateralized RVR ratio of >1.5-2.0 has predictive value for benefit from surgery.

RENAL CELL CARCINOMA (See Tumors)

RENAL TUBULAR ACIDOSIS
Type I (classic)
- URINE - pH not below 6.5.

•BLOOD - Non-anion-gap acidosis, hypokalemia.
•RADIOGRAPHY- Flat plate of abdomen may show nephrocalcinosis.

Type II (proximal)
•URINE - pH low, Fanconi's Syndrome common.
•BLOOD - Non-anion-gap acidosis and hypokalemia.

Type IV
•URINE - pH usually low.
•BLOOD - Non-anion gap acidosis, with elevation of BUN and
    Creatinine hyperkalemia often present.

RENAL VEIN THROMBOSIS
•URINE - Hematuria, proteinuria.
•RENAL ULTRASOUND - Widened renal vein with clots within the
    vein.
•CT SCAN - widened renal vein with clots within the vein.
•RENAL VENOGRAPHY - Typically visualizes the clot and point of
    obstruction.

SIADH (See Diabetes Insipidus)

SIMPLE CYST
•I.V.P. with NEPHROTOMOGRAM - Splaying or distortion of collection
    systems suggests a space occupying lesion. Nephrotomogram
    may show a cystic mass with a sharply defined border.
•ULTRASOUND - An area of decreased echogenicity may be seen.
•CYST BIOPSY - Bloody aspirate and abnormal cytology suggest
    malignancy.
•CT SCAN - Typically shows cysts.

SYSTEMIC LUPUS ERYTHEMATOSUS (SLE) (See SLE in Rheumatology Section)
•URINE- Proteinuria, hematuria and pyuria often present.
•KIDNEY BIOPSY - May show mesangial, membranous, focal or
    diffuse proliferative glomerulonephritis.

THROMBOTIC THROMBOCYTOPENIC PURPURA.
BLOOD, URINE, KIDNEY BIOPSY - Often similar to Hemolytic Uremic
    Syndrome (differentiation is clinical).

URIC ACID NEPHROPATHY
- BLOOD - BUN and creatinine may be elevated. Serum uric acid typically greater than 15 mg/dl.
- URINE - Spot uric acid and urine creatinine ratio usually greater than 1. Fractional excretion of uric acid may be high (>50%).

URINARY TRACT INFECTION
- URINALYSIS- Pyuria, bacteruria and often microscopic hematuria Leukocyte Esterase and Nitrates often positive.
- URINE CULTURE - Usually positive often with gram negative rods.

VESICO-URETERAL REFLUX
(See Reflux Nephropathy.)

VITAMIN D RESISTANT RICKETS
(FAMILIAL HYPOPHOSPHATEMIA)
- URINE - Phosphate/creatinine clearance ratio typically elevated. Calcium decreased.
- BLOOD - Hypophosphatemia (Calcium and PTH normal), alkaline phosphatase may be increased.
- SKELETAL FILMS - Shortened and rachitic long bones may be seen, with retarded bone age.

WILM'S TUMOR   (See TUMORS)

NEPHROLOGY REFERENCES

ACUTE INTERSTITIAL NEPHRITIS
1. Kleinknecht, D., Vanhille, P., Morel-Maroger, L., et al.: Acute interstitial nephritis due to drug hypersensitivity: An up to date review with a report of 19 cases. *Adv. Nephrol.* 1983; 12:277-308.
2. Nolan, C. R., Anger, M. S., Kelleher, S. P.: Eosinophiluria - a new method of detection and definition of the clinical spectrum. *N. E. J. M.* 1986; 315:1516-1519.

ACUTE TUBULAR NECROSIS
1. Miller, T. R., Anderson, R. J., Linas, S. L., et . al.: Urinary diagnostic indices in acute renal failure. *Ann. Intern. Med.* 1978; 89:47-50.
2. Corwin, H. L., Schreiber, M. J., Fang, L. S.: Fractional excretion of sodium: exceptions to its diagnostic value. *Arch. Intern. Med.* 1985; 145:108-112.

ALPORT'S SYNDROME
1. Grunfeld, J. P. The clinical spectrum of hereditary nephritis.: *Kidney Int.* 1981; 19:86-102.
2. Gubler, M., Levy, M., Broyer, M., et. al.: Alport's Syndrome. A report of 58 cases and a review of the literature. *Am. J. Med.* 1981; 70:493.

AMYLOIDOSIS
1. Vaamonde, C.A., Pardo, V.: Multiple myeloma and amyloidosis. In Schrier, R.W., Gottschalk, C.W. Disease of the Kidney, 4th Ed. Boston,
Little, Brown and Comp. 1988, pp 2455-2472.

ANALGESIC NEPHROPATHY (PAPILLARY NECROSIS)
1. Weber, M., Kuzz, P., Schild, H., et. al.: Comparison of conventional radiology, computed tomography and sonography in recognising papillary calcification in Analgesic Nephropathy. *Dial. and Trans.* 1987; 16:332-333.
2. Eknoyan, G.: Analgesic nephrotoxicity and renal papillary necrosis. *Semin. Nephrol.* 1984; 4:65-76.

BARTTER'S SYNDROME
1. Gill, J. R., Bartter, F. C.: Evidence for a prostaglandin independent defect in chloride reabsorption in the loop of Henle as a proximal cause of Bartter's Syndrome. *Am. J. Med.* 1978; 65:766-772.

2. Dunn, M. J. Prostaglandin and Bartter's syndrome. *Kidney Int.* 1981; 19:86-102.

BERGER'S DISEASE (IgA NEPHROPATHY)
1. Wyatt, R. J., Julian, B. A., Bhatena, D.B , et. al.: IgA Nephropathy: Presentation, clinical course and prognosis in children and adults. *Am. J. Kidney Dis.* 1984; 4:192-200.
2. D'Amico, G., Imbasciali, E., Belgioioso, G., et. al.: Idiopathic IgA mesangial Nephropathy Clinical and histological study of 376 patients. *Medicine* 1985; 64:49-60.

CALCULI
1. Rous, S. N. (ed). Evaluation of Urolithiasis patient. Stone disease: diagnosis and management. Grunne and Stralton. 1987.
2. Saklayen, M., Mital, C. Nephrolithiasis. In Barnes, H. V. (ed). Clinical Medicine: Selected problems with clinicopathologic correlation. Chicago, Medical Year Book Publishers. 1988.

CANCER (KIDNEY)
1. Garnick, M.B., Richie, J.P. Primary neoplasms of the kidney and renal pelvis. In Schrier, R.W., Gottschalk, C.W. Disease of the Kidney, 4th Ed. Boston, Little, Brown and Comp. 1988, pp 863-887.
2. O'Reilly, P. H., et. al Renal imaging: a comparison of radionuclide, ultrasound and CT scanning in investigation of renal space occupying lesion. *Br. Med. J.* 1981; 282:943.
3. Richie, J. P., Garnick, M. B., Seltzer, S., et. al.: Computerized tomography scan for diagnosis and staging of renal cell carcinoma. *J. Urol.* 1983; 129:1114.

DIABETES INSIPIDUS
1. Berl, T., Anderson, R. J., McDonald, K. M., et. al.: Clinical disorder of water metabolism. *Kidney Int.* 1976; 10:117.
2. Berl, T., Schrier, R. W.: Disorder of water metabolism. In Schrier, R. W. (ed), Renal and electrolyte disorders, 3rd Ed. Boston, Little, Brown and Comp. 1986.

FABRY'S DISEASE
1. Desnick, R. J., Allen, K. Y., Desnick, S. J., et . al.: Fabry's disease: enzymatic diagnosis of hemizygotes and heterozygotes. *J. Lab. Clin. Med.* 1973; 81:157.
2. Farraggiana, T., Churg, J., Grishman, E., et. al.: Light and electron microscopic histochemistry of Fabry's Disease. *Am. J. Pathol.* 1981; 103:247.

GLOMERULONEPHRITIS

1. Glassock, R. J., et. al.: Primary Glomerular disease. The Kidney. 3rd edition. Brenner and Rector (eds). W. B. Saunders 1987.
2. Savage, C. S., Winearls, C. G., Evans, D. J., et. al.: Microscopic Polyarteritis: presentation, pathology and prognosis. *Q. J. Med.* 1985; 56:467-483.

POST STREPTOCOCCAL GLOMERULONEPHRITIS

1. Rodriguez-Iturbe, B.: Epidemic Post-streptococcal glomerulonephritis. *Kidney Int.* 1984; 25:129.
2. Bergner-Rabinowitz, S., Fleiderman, S., Ferne, M.: The new streptozyme test for streptococcal antibodies.*Clin. Pediatr.* 1975; 14:804.

GOODPASTURE'S SYNDROME

1. Sevekjian, H., Knight, H., Weinman, E.: The spectrum of renal disease associated with antibasement membrane antibodies. *Arch. Intern. Med.* 1980; 140:79.
2. Savage, C., Pusey, C., Bowman, C., et. al.: Antiglomerular basement membrane antibody mediated diseases in British Isle 1980-84. *Br. Med. J.*1985; 292:301-304.

LEAD NEPHROPATHY

1. Wedeen, R. P., Mallik, D. K., Batuman, V.: Detection and treatment of occupational lead nephropathy. *Arch. Intern. Med.* 1979; 139:53-57.
2. Bennet, W. M. Lead Nephropathy. *Kidney Int.* 1985; 28:212-220.

LIDDLE'S SYNDROME

1. Rodriguez, J. A., Bigleeri, E. G., Scharmbelan, M.: Pseudohyper-aldosteronism with tubular resistance to mineralocorticoid hormone. *Clin. Res.* 1981; 29:567A.

MEDULLARY CYSTIC DISEASE

1. Straus, M. B.: Clinical and pathological aspects of cystic disease of the renal medulla: an analysis of 18 cases. *Ann. Intern. Med.* 1962; 57:373.

MEDULLARY SPONGE KIDNEY

1. Harrison, A. R, Rose, G. A.: Medullary Sponge Kidney. *Urol. Res.* 1979; 7:197.

MYELOMA KIDNEY
1. Rota, S., Mougenol, B., Baudouin, B., et. al.: Multiple Myeloma and severe renal failure: a clinicopathologic study of outcome and prognosis in 34 patients. *Medicine* 1987; 66:127-137.

MYOGLOBINURIA
1. Honda, N., Kurokawa, K.: Acute renal failure and rhabdomyolysis. *Kidney Int.* 1983; 23:888-898.

NEPHROTIC SYNDROME
1. Schnaper, H.W., Robson, A.M.: Nephrotic syndrome: minimal change disease, focal glomerulosclerosis and related disorders. In Schrier, R.W., Gottschalk, C.W. Disease of the Kidney, 4th Ed. Boston, Little, Brown and Comp. 1988, pp 1949-1986.

OBSTRUCTIVE UROPATHY
1. Malave, S. R., Neiman, H. L., Spies, S. M., et . al.: Diagnosis of hydronephrosis: comparison of radionuclide scanning and sonography. *A. J. R.* 1980; 135:1179.
2. Scheible, W., Talner, L. B.: Gray scale ultrasound and the genito-urinary tract: a review of clinical applications. *Radiol. Clin. N. Am.* 1978; 17:281.

ORTHOSTATIC PROTEINURIA
1. Kassirer, J.P., Harrington, J.T.: Laboratory evaluation of renal failure. In Schrier, R.W., Gottschalk, C.W. Disease of the Kidney, 4th Ed. Boston, Little, Brown and Comp. 1988, pp 427-428.

PAPILLARY NECROSIS
1. Weber, M., Kuzz, P., Schild, H., et. al.: Comparison of conventional radiology, computed tomography and sonography in recognising papillary calcification in Analgesic Nephropathy. *Dial. and Trans.* 1987; 16:332-333.
2. Eknoyan, G.: Analgesic nephrotoxicity and renal papillary necrosis. *Semin. Nephrol* 1984; 4:65-76.

POLYCYSTIC KIDNEY DISEASE
1. Milutinovic, J., Philips, L. A., Bryant, J. I., et. al.: Autosomal dominant polycystic kidney disease: early diagnosis and data for genetic counseling. *Lancet* 1980; 1:1203.
2. Levine, E., Grantham, J. J.: The role of computed tomography in the evaluation of adult polycystic kidney disease. *Am. J. Kidney Dis.* 1981; 1:99.

PRERENAL AZOTEMIA
1. Levi, M., Rowe, J.W. Aging and the Kidney. In Schrier, R.W., Gottschalk, C.W. Disease of the Kidney, 4th Ed. Boston, Little, Brown and Comp. 1988, pp 2672-2673.

PYELONEPHRITIS
1. Pollack, H. M.: Laboratory techniques for detection of urinary tract infection and assessment of value. *Am. J. Med* 1983; 75(1B):79.

RAPIDLY PROGRESSIVE GLOMERULONEPHRITIS
1. Atkins, R.C., Thompson, N.M. Rapidly progressive glomerulo-nephritis. In Schrier, R.W., Gottschalk, C.W. Disease of the Kidney, 4th Ed. Boston, Little, Brown and Comp. 1988, pp 1903-21.

RENAL ARTERY STENOSIS
1. Hillman, B.J., Brewer, M.L. Diagnostic and therapeutic imaging of the renal circulation: film-screen arteriography, digital subtraction angiography, and percutaneous angioplasty and embolization. In Schrier, R.W., Gottschalk, C.W. Disease of the Kidney, 4th Ed. Boston, Little, Brown and Comp. 1988, pp. 497-517.

RENAL TUBULAR ACIDOSIS (RTA)
1. Battle, D.: Renal tubular acidosis. *Med. Clin. N. Am.* 1983;67:89.
2. Battle, D., Kurtzman, N. A. Distal renal tubular acidosis. *Am. J. Kidney Dis.* 1982; 1:328-344.

RENAL VEIN THROMBOSIS
1. Llach, F., Papper, S., Massry, S. G.: The clinical spectrum of renal vein thrombosis: acute and chronic. *Am. J. Med.* 1980; 69:819-822.
2. Avashti, P. S., Green, E. R., Scholler, C., et. al.: Non-invasive diagnosis of renal vein thrombosis by ultrasonic echo doppler flowmetry. *Kidney Int.* 1983; 23:882-887.

SIADH
1. Berl, T., Anderson, R. J., McDonald, K. M., et. al.: Clinical disorder of water metabolism. *Kidney Int.* 1976; 10:117.
2. Berl, T., Schrier, R. W.: Disorder of water metabolism. In Schrier, R.W., Gottschalk, C.W. Disease of the Kidney, 4th Ed. Boston, Little, Brown. 1988.

SIMPLE CYST

1. Demas, B.E., Hricak, H.: Computed tomography and magnetic resonance imaging. In Schrier, R.W., Gottschalk, C.W. Disease of the Kidney, 4th Ed. Boston, Little, Brown. 1988, pp 481-485.

URIC ACID NEPHROPATHY

1. Emmerson, B.T., Hyperuricemia, gout, and the kidney.: In Schrier, R.W., Gottschalk, C.W. Disease of the Kidney, 4th Ed. Boston, Little, Brown. 1988, pp 2481-2506.

VESICO-URETERAL REFLUX (VUR)

1. Conway, J. J. Radionuclide cystography.: *Contrib. to Nephrol.* 1984; 39:1.
2. Hodson,C. Reflux nephropathy. *Med. Clin. N. Am.* 1978;62:1201.

VITAMIN D RESISTANT RICKETS (V.D.R.R.)

1. Stickler, G. B., Beabout, J. W., Riggs, B. C., et. al.: Vitamin D resistant rickets: clinical experience with 61 typical familial hypophosphatemic patients and atypical non-familial cases. *Mayo. Clin. Proc.* 1970; 45:197.

WEGNER'S GRANULOMATOSIS

1. Pinching, A. J., Lockwood, C. M., Pussel, B. A., et. al.: Wegner's granulomatosis: observations on 18 patients with severe renal disease. *Q. J. Med.* 1983; 52:435-460.2.Savage, C. S., Winearls, Jones, S., et. al.: Prospective study of radio-immunoassay for antibodies against neutrophil cytoplasm in diagnosis of systemic vasculitis. *Lancet* 1987; 1:1389-1393.

WILM'S TUMOR

1. Henig, R., Kinser, J.: Ultrasonic diagnosis of Wilm's tumor. *Am. J. Roentgenol.* 1973; 117:119.

NEUROLOGY

The number, types and priority of tests ordered must be individualized for each patient, consequently the tests listed for each disease in this chapter are not prioritized and are not exhaustive.

CANCER (BRAIN)
CANCER of BRAIN or SPINAL CORD
•CT SCAN/MRI - May show mass lesion.

MENINGEAL CARCINOMATOSIS/LEUKEMIA
•LUMBAR PUNCTURE - CSF cytology for malignant cells.

SPINAL CORD TUMORS
•EMG - May indicate level of tumor.
•RADIOGRAPHY -
  -Spine radiograph: may show destruction of vertebral body or
    pedicle or enlargement of intervertebral formina.
  -Myelography: subdural, extramedullary (cup-shaped)
    obstruction may be seen.
  -MRI of spine typically shows cord mass.
  -Bone Scan may show area of increased uptake prior to bone
    destruction.

CERBROVASCULAR DISEASE
ISCHEMIC STROKES (THROMBO-EMBOLIC)
Including TIA, Reversible Ischemic Neurologic Deficit (RIND) and
  Lacunar strokes.
•CT SCAN/MRI - May show location and presence or absence of
  hemorrhage. MRI more sensitive in white matter strokes, deep
  lacunar, brain stem and cerebellar strokes.
•Neck and Cerebral Circulation:
  Ultrasound may show obstruction of carotids.
  Digital Subtraction Angiography (Intra-arterial) may show
    obstruction or stenosis in the carotids and major intracerebral
    vessels. Cerebral Angiography may show obstruction and
    lesion in the carotids and major intracerebral vessels.
•Cardiac Evaluation
  Echocardiography may demonstrate clot or vegetation in the
    atria or ventricle.

SUBARACHNOID HEMORRHAGE
•CT SCAN - Without contrast may show blood in basal cisterns and
  fissures.
  With contrast may show aneurysm or arteriovenous malformation
  (CT scan cannot entirely rule out subarachnoid hemorrhage).

- LUMBAR PUNCTURE - When CT is negative but clinical picture suggests subarachnoid hemorrhage. CSF may show increased RBC or xanthochromia.
- ECG - Non-specific ST-T wave changes, arrhythmias.
- BLOOD - Hyponatremia may be seen due to Syndrome of Inappropriate ADH. Bleeding disorders may cause subarachnoid hemorrhage or intracerebral hematoma.
- CEREBRAL ANGIOGRAPHY - Definitive test to identify aneurysm or arterio-venous malformation.
- MRI - May demonstrate flow deficit in arterio-venous malformation and aneurysms.

ANEURYSM
   (See -Subarachnoid hemorrhage).

ARTERIOVENOUS MALFORMATION
   (See - Subarachnoid hemorrhage.

INTRACEREBRAL HEMATOMA
   (See - Subarachnoid Hemorrhage)

DEMENTIAS
ALZHEIMER'S DISEASE
- CT SCAN - Demonstrates brain atrophy.
- Consider the laboratory evaluation of other causes of dementia.

CRUETZFELD JAKOB DISEASE
- EEG - Characteristic sharp and slow waves.
- LUMBAR PUNCTURE - CSF is usually normal.
- BRAIN BIOPSY - rarely done, shows characteristic spongiform encephalopathy.

HUNTINGTON'S DISEASE
- CT SCAN/MRI - Selective caudate atrophy may be seen.

NORMAL PRESSURE HYDROCEPHALUS
- CT SCAN/MRI - Enlarged third ventricle with normal fourth ventricle.
- ISOTOPE CISTERNOGRAPHY - Communicating hydrocephalus with obliteration of the sub-arachnoid space.

VASCULAR DEMENTIA (MULTI-INFARCT, BINGSWANGER'S)
•MRI - May show multiple small areas of infarction.
•Neck Vessels - See Cerebrovascular.

WILSON'S DISEASE (HEPATO-LENTICULAR DEGENERATION
(See Gastroenterology Section - Cirrhosis).

DEMYELINATING & DYSMYELINATING DISEASES
ACUTE DISSEMINATED ENCEPHALOMYELITIS
(ACUTE HEMORRHAGIC LEUCOENCEPHALOPATHY)
•LUMBAR PUNCTURE - CSF: increased blood cells and protein.
•CT SCAN/MRI - Multifocal lesions with/without mass effect.

CENTRAL PONTINE MYELINOLYSIS
•MRI - Lesions in pontine base, scattered lesions in white matter.

MULTIPLE SCLEROSIS
•LUMBAR PUNCTURE - CSF:Increased lymphocytes during
  exacerbation, total protein normal or slightly increased, IgG
  increased in 60%, Oligoclonal protein bands present in 80-90%,
  Myelin basic protein increased during active disease.

•EVOKED RESPONSES - Visual, brain stem and somatosensory.
  May show subclinical ("silent") deficits in visual or auditory
  pathways, or spinal cord

•MRI - May show plaques.

PROGRESSIVE MULTIFOCAL LEUCOENCEPHALOPATHY
•CT SCAN/MRI - May show multifocal white matter lesions.
•LUMBAR PUNCTURE - CSF: Lymphocytic pleocytosis.
•BIOPSY - Brain: there is characteristic histopathology giant
  astrocytes,gliosis and perivascular inflammation. Electron
  microscopy may show Papova virus.

EPILEPSY: SEIZURE DISORDER
•EEG - May show paroxysmal focal or generalized spikes and
  waves.
•CT / MRI - May show structural lesions.

- **LUMBAR PUNCTURE** - May show evidence of meningitis or encephalitis.
- **BLOOD** - Chemistries and drug screen may show toxic / metabolic etiologies of seizures.

METABOLIC DISEASES
ACUTE INTERMITTENT PORPHYRIA
- **URINE** - Watson-Schwartz test: typically shows increased porphobilinogen, porphyrins and delta aminolevulinic acid.

LESCH-NYHAN SYNDROME (Disorder of purine metabolism)
- **BLOOD** - Increased uric acid is typical.
- Increased Hypoxanthine-guanine phosphoribosyl transferase in RBC's and cultured fibroblasts.

LYSOSOMAL STORAGE DISEASES
TAY-SACHS DISEASE (GM_2 GANGLIOSIDOSIS)
- **BLOOD** - Decreased hexosaminidase in serum and leukocytes. Prenatal diagnosis made by detecting enzyme deficiency in cultured fibroblasts from amniocentesis.

METACHROMATIC LEUKODYSTROPHY (disorder of glycolipid metabolism)
- **BLOOD** - Decreased Aryl Sulphatase A in serum, leukocytes and cultured fibroblasts.

PHENYLKETONURIA (disorder of amino acid metabolism)
- **BLOOD** - Increased phenylalanine. Reduced phenylalanine hydroxylase.
- **URINE** - Increased phenylpyruvic acid.

REYES SYNDROME
- **BLOOD** - Increased liver function tests and ammonia may be seen.
- **CT SCAN** - Diffuse cerebral edema may be present.
- **LUMBAR PUNCTURE** - Increased pressure, but normal CSF.

SUBACUTE COMBINED DEGENERATION
- **BLOOD** - Anemia, increased MCV is typical. Decreased serum folate and B_{12} may be seen.
- **EMG** - may show peripheral neuropathy.

NEUROMUSCULAR DISEASES
- MUSCLE ENZYMES -CPK, AST, LDH, aldolase may be elevated.
- URINE - Myoglobinuria may be seen in acute severe muscle disease.
- EMG - Shows myopathic potentials.
- MUSCLE BIOPSY - Light and electron microscopy and histochemistry may show pathologic changes (variable) depending upon etiology.

GENETIC METABOLIC MYOPATHIES
- MUSCLE HISTOCHEMISTRY and ENZYME ASSAYS - May show specific muscle enzyme deficiency or abnormal metabolite.
- MUSCLE BIOPSY and ELECTRON MICROSCOPY - May show characteristic pattern of specific myopathy.

MOTOR NEURON DISEASE (AMYOTROPHIC LATERAL SCLEROSIS)
- EMG - Typically shows widespread anterior horn involvement in extremities and cranial muscles.
- MUSCLE BIOPSY - May show neurogenic atrophy.

MYASTHENIA GRAVIS
- Neuro-muscular Junction Deficit abnormal, demonstrated by abnormal Tensilon, Neostigmine or Curare test.
- EMG - Shows decreasing amplitude with repetitive stimulation.
- BLOOD - Acetyl choline receptor antibodies (present in 70-85%), thyroid function tests may be abnormal in 10% of myasthenics.
- CHEST CT SCAN / X-RAY - may show thymic enlargement.

MYASTHENIC SYNDROME (EATON-LAMBERT)
- EMG - Shows increasing amplitude with repetitive stimulation.

RADICULOPATHIES and HERNIATED DISC (NECK and BACK PAIN)
- RADIOGRAPHY CT Scan of spine: may show impingement on spinal cord or nerve root not as useful for cervical spine, better for lumbar discs. MRI: extremely sensitive for cervical spine and myelopathy may help demonstrate anatomy of lesion. Myelography may also help define the anatomy of the lesion in some cases.

NEUROPATHIES (INCLUDING PERIPHERAL NERVE ENTRAPMENT)

- •EMG AND NERVE CONDUCTION VELOCITIES - May show conduction: block, slowing or neuropathic potentials.
- •LUMBAR PUNCTURE - May show elevated protein.
- •SURAL NERVE BIOPSY - May show vasculitis or demyelination.

NEUROLOGY REFERENCES

CANCER (BRAIN)
1. Shapiro, W. R. Intracranial Neoplasms. In Rosenberg, R. N., Grossman, R. G. (eds): The Clinical Neurosciences. New York, Churchill Livingstone. 1983, pp 233-283.

CEREBROVASCULAR DISEASE
1. Millikan, C. H., McDowell, F., Easton, J. D. Stroke. Philadelphia, Lee Febiger. 1987.

DEMENTIAS
1. Hutton, J. T. (ed). Dementia: Neurologic Clinics of North America. 1987.

DEMYELINATING DISEASES
1. Weiner, H. L., Hufler, D. A. Multiple Sclerosis. In Appel, S. H. (ed): Current Neurology, vol. 6. Chicago, Year Book Medical Publishers. 1986, pp 123-151.

EPILEPSY
1. Mathew, T. Seizure Disorders. In Barnes, H. V. (ed): Clinical Medicine: Selected Problems with pathophysiologic corelations. Chicago, Medical Year Book Publishers. 1988, pp 719-725

METABOLIC DISEASE
1. Ravel, R. Clinical Laboratory Medicine, 4th Ed. Chicago, Medical Year Book Publishers. 1984.

NEUROMUSCULAR DISEASES
1. Baker, A. B., Joynt , R. J.(eds). Clinical Neurology. Philadelphia, Harper and Row. 1987.

PULMONARY

The number, types and priority of tests ordered must be individualized for each patient, consequently the tests listed for each disease in this chapter are not prioritized and are not exhaustive.

ADULT RESPIRATORY DISTRESS SYNDROME (ARDS)
- ARTERIAL BLOOD GAS - PaO_2 decreased, PCO_2 usually normal.
- CHEST RADIOGRAPH - Diffuse "fluffy"infiltrates; "White Out".
- Increased Intrapulmonary shunting with increased A-a PO_2 difference. (A-a difference = alveolar PAO_2- arterial PaO_2).

ALLERGIC BRONCHOPULMONARY ASPERGILLOSIS
- SPUTUM - *Aspergillus* fungus may be seen on microscopy.
- SKIN REACTION to *Aspergillus* - immediate.
- BLOOD - IgE elevated, eosinophilia and *Aspergillus* precipitins elevated.
- CHEST RADIOGRAPH - Pulmonary infiltrates; central bronchiectasis.

ASPERGILLOMA
- SPUTUM - *Aspergillus* fungus may be seen on microscopy.
- BLOOD - Increased *Aspergillus* precipitins.
- CHEST RADIOGRAPH - Moveable intracavitary mass surrounded on its superior surface by a crescent of air (Monod's sign) may be seen.

ASPERGILLOSIS (OPPORTUNISTIC PULMONARY)
- SPUTUM, BLOOD, URINE, CSF CULTURES are rarely positive.
- TRANSTRACHEAL ASPIRATION - May have positive cultures.
- BRONCHOSCOPY (with brushing and transbronchial biopsy). May show invasion of lung tissue.

ASTHMA
- SPUTUM wet mount - Often with spiral casts, eosinophils, Charcot-Leyden crystals.
- PULMONARY FUNCTION TESTS - Reversible airway obstruction by bronchodilator or positive methacholine challenge.
- BLOOD - IgE elevated, eosinophilia.
- CHEST RADIOGRAPH - May show hyperinflation.
- SKIN TESTS - May have positive wheal and flare reaction to specific allergens.
- ARTERIAL BLOOD GAS - May be consistent with obstructive airway disease.

ATELECTASIS
- CHEST RADIOGRAPH - If mild: discrete areas of increased density may be seen in lung fields. If massive: Entire lung may be collapsed with hyperlucent area surrounding the lung parenchyma.

BRONCHITIS (CHRONIC)
- SPUTUM - Increased volume (criteria = increased daily sputum production for 3 months during two consecutive years), mucopurulent. May have sputum eosinophilia in asthmatic bronchitis.
- ECG - May show right axis deviation, right ventricular hypertrophy.
- PULMONARY FUNCTION TESTS - Decreased FEV, FEV_1/FVC < 75%.
- ARTERIAL BLOOD GAS - May show mild to moderate widening of A-a gradient, hypoxemia, hypercapnia, respiratory acidosis.
- BLOOD - May have elevated hematocrit and eosinophilia in asthmatic bronchitis.
- CHEST RADIOGRAPH - Normal or flat hemidiaphragms, may have increased AP chest diameter and increased lung markings in periphery, heart size large in cor pulmonale.

CANCER (LUNG)
- SPUTUM CYTOLOGY - Neoplastic cells may be seen.
- CHEST RADIOGRAPH - PA and lateral may show a mass.
- BRONCHOSCOPY - Brushings, segmental washings and biopsy may demonstrate neoplastic cells.
- NEEDLE ASPIRATION - May show neoplastic cells.
- OPEN BIOPSY - May show neoplastic cells.

SQUAMOUS CELL
- BLOOD - Calcium, PTH and occasionally ACTH and HCG may be elevated.
- CHEST RADIOGRAPH - Lesion is usually central in location.
- BIOPSY - May see keratin pearls in well differentiated cancer.

SMALL CELL CARCINOMA INCLUDING OAT CELL
- BLOOD - May have elevated ACTH, Calcitonin, ADH, and HCG.
- CHEST RADIOGRAPH - Usually the lesion is central in location, mediastinal spread is common at the time of diagnosis.
- BIOPSY - Small dark staining cells with sparse cytoplasm.

ADENOCARCINOMA
•BLOOD - May have elevation of GH and HCG.
•CHEST RADIOGRAPH - Lesion is usually peripheral in location.
•BIOPSY - Glandular structures and excess mucous staining are
    present.

LARGE CELL CARCINOMA
•BLOOD - May have elevated GH and HCG.
•CHEST RADIOGRAPH - Lesion may be in any location.
•BIOPSY - Large, polygonal vesicular cells are seen.

COPD (CHRONIC OBSTRUCTIVE PULMONARY DISEASE) (SEE BRONCHITIS AND EMPHYSEMA)

ALLERGIC ANGIITIS AND GRANULOMATOSIS (CHURG-STRAUSS SYNDROME)
•BLOOD - May have eosinophilia, elevated IgE, anemia, elevated
    ESR.
•BIOPSY - Usually demonstrates eosinophilic, necrotizing,
    extravascular granulomas and necrotizing vasculitis of arterioles
    and venules.

CYSTIC FIBROSIS
•SWEAT TEST- By Pilocarpine iontophoresis shows sweat chloride
    greater than 60 meq/L.
•CHEST RADIOGRAPH - Bronchiectasis with signs of COPD:
    flattened diaphragm, increased AP chest diameter, decreased
    vascular markings, bullae and blebs, heart size normal or small,
    or hyperinflation.
•SPUTUM - Often contains mucoid strains of *pseudomonas* .
•SECRETIN or CCK-PZ TESTS - Usually shows inpaired production
    of bicarbonate or pancreatic enzymes, respectively.
•BLOOD - Trypsin levels often decreased as disease progresses.

EMBOLISM (SEE PULMONARY EMBOLISM)

EMPHYSEMA
•SPUTUM - Clear, mucoid.
•PULMONARY FUNCTION TESTS - Decreased FEV_1, FEV_1/FVC
    ratio, and DLCO.

•BLOOD - Mild to moderate widening of A-a PO_2 gradient, Alpha-1-antitrypsin - may be decreased.
•CHEST RADIOGRAPH - May show flattened diaphragm, increased AP chest diameter, decreased vascular markings, bullae and blebs, heart size normal or small, hyperinflation.

HISTOPLASMOSIS
ACUTE
•BLOOD - Elevated Histoplama titers (complement fixation test).
•CHEST RADIOGRAPH - May show patchy infiltrate with hilar adenopathy.

CHRONIC
•SPUTUM - May see fungus.
•CHEST RADIOGRAPH - Typically an upper lobe cavitary disease.

DISSEMINATED (typically immunocompromised patients)
•BLOOD - Histoplama titers may be negative.
•CHEST RADIOGRAPH - Abnormalities present in half of cases shows discrete nodules or miliary pattern.

IDIOPATHIC PULMONARY FIBROSIS (HAMMAN-RICH SYNDROME)
•PULMONARY FUNCTION TESTS - Decreased vital capacity, and total lung capacity, normal or increased. FEV_1/FVC ratio, decreased DLCO.
•BLOOD - May have Rheumatoid Factor.
•ARTERIAL BLOOD GAS - Mild hypoxemia-worsens with exercise, pCO_2 mildly reduced, also worsens with exercise.
•CHEST RADIOGRAPH - May show diffuse reticular, nodular or reticulonodular patterns, honey-combing.

IMMOTILE CILIA SYNDROME
•Sperm motility is decreased.
•ELECTRON MICROSCOPY - Absence of dynein arms or radial spokes in cilia, may confirm the diagnosis.
•SCREENING TEST - Scrapings or nasal epithelium biopsy if immediately observed for ciliary beat demonstrates a decrease in ciliary motion.

KARTAGENER'S SYNDROME
•CHEST RADIOGRAPH - Bronchiectasis. Situs inversus sometimes present.
•SINUS FILMS - Sinusitis often seen.

YOUNG'S SYNDROME
•AZOSPERMIA.
•CHEST RADIOGRAPH - May show repeated pulmonary infection.
•SINUS FILMS - May show chronic sinusitis.

MESOTHELIOMA, PLEURAL
•CHEST RADIOGRAPH - Occasional pleural effusion and Pleural mass.
•THORACENTESIS - Pleural fluid serous or blood stained, occasionally neoplastic cells may be found on cytologic examination.
•BIOPSY - Open pleural may demonstrate neoplastic cells or tissue.
•CT SCAN - Pleural mass (masses tend to line or encase the lung).

PNEUMOCONIOSIS
ASBESTOSIS
•SPUTUM - Decreased volume and presence of dumbbell-shaped asbestosis needles in clusters may be seen.
•CHEST RADIOGRAPH - Small linear opacities in lower lung fields (initial abnormality). Lung volume decreased, pleural plaques (often visible along the diaphragm).
•PULMONARY FUNCTION TESTS - May show the restrictive pattern of pulmonary fibrosis (see Idiopathic Pulmonary Fibrosis).

COAL WORKERS
•CHEST RADIOGRAPH - Early stage: small, irregular opacities (reticular pattern). Prolonged exposure: small, rounded, regular opacities, 1-5mm in diameter (nodular pattern).

SILICOSIS
•CHEST RADIOGRAPH - Egg shell lymph node calcification. Simple Silicosis: small, rounded opacities or nodules. Complicated Silicosis: nodules become larger and coalescent.

•PULMONARY FUNCTION TESTS -Normal in simple silicosis.
Restrictive, obstructive and mixed abnormalities as disease
progresses.

BERYLLIUM
•CHEST RADIOGRAPH - Acute fulminant form: bronchiolitis,
pneumonia and pulmonary edema. Chronic diffuse
granulomatous pneumonitis may progress to pulmonary fibrosis,
and hilar nodes may calcify.
•PULMONARY FUNCTION TESTS - Normal or restrictive disease
changes.
•TISSUE and URINE - Beryllium positive (urine concentration may
correlate with disease activity).

TALC
•CHEST RADIOGRAPH - Interstitial fibrosis and restrictive disease.
•PULMONARY FUNCTION TESTS - May be consistent with restrictive
disease.
(See Idiopathic Pulmonary Fibrosis).

IRON
•CHEST RADIOGRAPH - Radiodense collections may be seen.
•PULMONARY FUNCTION TESTS - Usually normal.
FIBERGLASS
•CHEST RADIOGRAPH - Usually normal, occasionally small
opacities.
•PULMONARY FUNCTION TESTS - Usually normal.

PNEUMONIA
General
•SPUTUM - Gram stain and culture may identify the organism.
•BLOOD - Elevated WBC count, positive cultures (2 cultures from
different sights is usually adequate).
•THORACENTESIS (if pleural effusion) - Gram stain and culture may
identify organism.

S. PNEUMONIA
•CHEST RADIOGRAPH - Consolidation (classically lobar) may be
seen.

S. PYOGENES (RARE)
•CHEST RADIOGRAPH - Pleural effusion/empyema may be seen.

S. AUREUS
•CHEST RADIOGRAPH - Usually bronchopneumonia with possible cavitation.

NEISERRIA MENINGITIDIS
•CHEST RADIOGRAPH - Patchy alveolar consolidation may be seen.

H. INFLUENZA
•CHEST RADIOGRAPH - Diffuse bronchopneumonia and pleural effusion may be seen.

KLEBSIELLA PNEUMONIA
•CHEST RADIOGRAPH - Upper lobe air space pneumonia *ie.* bulging fissure sign with cavitary spaces), abscess formation, and pleural effusion may be seen.

M. PNEUMONIA
•CHEST RADIOGRAPH - Segmental bronchopneumonia (Film usually worse than clinical findings), may be associated with pleural effusion.

VIRAL
•CHEST RADIOGRAPH - Patchy infiltrate may be seen.

Legionella
•SPUTUM - Immunofluorescent staining and culture may show the organism.
•CHEST RADIOGRAPH - Usually initially patchy infiltrate progressing to consolidation.

PNEUMOTHORAX
•CHEST RADIOGRAPH - Visceral pleural line visible. Tension pneumothorax: large amount of air in the affected hemithorax and contralateral shift of mediastinal structures.
•ARTERIAL BLOOD GAS - May show hypoxemia.

PULMONARY EMBOLUS
- ECG - Tachycardia is frequent. Acute pulmonary hypertension: Right axis deviation, peaked P waves, and ST-T wave changes of right heart strain pattern (S1, Q3, T3 pattern uncommon).
- CHEST RADIOGRAPH - Initially normal in most patients. If infarct occurs an infiltrate may be seen 12-24 hours later.
- V/Q SCAN (perfusion and ventilation scintiphotography) - Usually shows unmatched defects (no perfusion with normal ventilation).
- PULMONARY ANGIOGRAPHY - Shows abrupt vessel cutoff at embolus site, filling defects past the point of obstruction, and/or a delayed venous phase.
- OTHER DIAGNOSTIC STUDIES (for determination of deep venous thrombosis). Impedance Plethysmography: Typically shows venous outflow obstruction, highly sensitive to above knee obstruction, fails to show many below knee obstructions. Nuclear Venogram: Sensitive for below knee obstruction, requires 24 hours for definitive answer. Dye Venogram: Standard for showing venous outflow obstruction.

SARCOIDOSIS
- BLOOD - May show lymphocytopenia, occasional mild eosinophilia, increased ESR, hyperglobulinemia, increased angiotension converting enzyme, hypercalcemia, increased uric acid.
- CHEST RADIOGRAPH - May show bilateral hilar adenopathy, and/or parenchymal interstitial infiltration.
  - Stage I bilateral hilar adenopathy with no parenchymal abnormality.
  - Stage II bilateral hilar adenopathy with diffuse parenchymal changes.
  - Stage III diffuse parenchymal changes without hilar adenopathy.
- TRANSBRONCHIAL BIOPSY - Granulomatous inflammation.

TUBERCULOSIS
- PPD SKIN TEST (used as screening test) - skin test may be positive or negative in active disease.
- CHEST RADIOGRAPH - Upper lobe cavitary disease. Lower lobe involvement may be seen.
- SPUTUM - Acid fast bacillus.
- **Also see under Nephrology**

ADULT RESPIRATORY DISTRESS SYNDROME
1. Brandstetter, R. D.: The adult respiratory distress syndrome-1986. *Heart Lung* 1986; 15:155-164.
2. Petty, T. L.: Adult respiratory distress syndrome: definition and historical perspective. *Clin. Chest Med.* 1982; 3:3-7.
3. Bernard, G. R., Brigham, K. L.: The adult respiratory distress syndrome. *Annu. Rev. Med.* 1985; 36:195-205.
4. Bell, R. C., Coalson, J. J., Smith, J. D., Johanson, W. G. Jr.: Multiple organ system failure and infection in adult respiratory distress syndrome. *Ann. Intern. Med.* 1983; 99:293-298.
5. Petty, T. L., Fowler, A. A. 3d.: Another look at ARDS. *Chest* 1982; 82:98-104.

ALLERGIC BRONCHOPULMONARY ASPERGILLOSIS
1. Greenberger, P. A., Patterson, R.: Diagnosis and management of allergic bronchopulmonary aspergillosis. *Ann. Allergy* 1986; 56:444-448.
2. Rosenberg, M., Patterson, R., Mintzer, R., Cooper, B. J., Roberts, M., Harris, K. E.: Clinical and immunologic criteria for the diagnosis of allergic bronchopulmonary aspergillosis. *Ann. Intern. Med.* 1977; 86:405-414.
3. Glimp, R. A., Bayer, A. S.: Fungal pneumonias: Part 3. Allergic bronchopulmonary aspergillosis. *Chest* 1981; 80:85-94.

ASPERGILLOMA
1. Davis, D (ed). Aspergilloma and residual tuberculous cavities-the results of a resurvey. A report from the Research Committee of the British Thoracic and Tuberculosis Association. *Tubercle* 1970; 51:227-245.
2. Varkey, B., Rose, H. D.: Pulmonary aspergilloma. A rational approach to treatment. *Am. J. Med.* 1976; 61:626-631.

ASPERGILLOSIS (OPPORTUNISTIC PULMONARY)
1. Albelda, S. M., Talbot, G. H., Gerson, S. L., Miller, W. T., Cassileth, P. A.: Role of fiberoptic bronchoscopy in the diagnosis of invasive pulmonary aspergillosis in patients with acute leukemia. *Am. J. Med.* 1984; 76:1027-1034.
2. Herbert , P. A., Bayer, A. S.: Fungal pneumonia (part 4). Invasive pulmonary aspergillosis. *Chest.* 1981; 80:220-225.

ASTHMA
1. American Thoracic Society. Standards for the diagnosis and care of patients with chronic obstructive pulmonary disease (COPD) and asthma. *Am. Rev. Respir. Dis.* 1987; 136:225-244.
2. Jackson, L. K. Functional aspects of asthma. *Clin. Chest Med.* 1984; 5:573-587.
3. Boushey, H. A., Holtzman, M. J., Sheller, J. R., Nadel, J. A.: Bronchial hyperreactivity. *Am. Rev. Respir. Dis.* 1980; 121:389-413.

EMPHYSEMA (SEE BRONCHITIS)

ATELECTASIS
1. Fraser, R. G., Pare, J. A. Diagnosis of Diseases of the Chest, 2nd Ed. Philadelphia, W. B. Saunders Co. 1977, pp 379-410.
2. Felson, B. Chest Roentgenology. Philadelphia, W. B. Saunders Co. 1973, pp 92-133.

BRONCHITIS/EMPHYSEMA
1. American Thoracic Society. Standards for the diagnosis and care of patients with chronic obstructive pulmonary disease (COPD) and asthma. *Am. Rev. Respir. Dis* . 1987; 136:225-244.
2. Black, L. F.: Early diagnosis of chronic obstructive pulmonary disease. *Mayo. Clin. Proc* . 1982; 57:765-772.
3. Peto, R., Speizer, F. E., Cochrane, A. L., Moore, F., Fletcher, C. M., Tinker, C. M., et. al.: The relevance in adults of air-flow obstruction, but not mucus hypersecretion, to mortality from chronic lung disease. *Am. Rev. Respir. Dis.* 1983; 128:491-500.
4. Bulter, C.: Bronchitis and emphysema. *Semin. Respir. Med.* 1982; 4:86-92.

CANCER (LUNG)
1. Skillrud, D. M., Offord, K. P., Miller, R. D.: Higher risk of lung cancer in chronic obstructive pulmonary disease. A prospective, matched, controlled study. *Ann. Intern. Med.* 1986; 105:503-507.
2. Carr, D. T (ed).: Cancer of the lung. Part 1. *Semin. Respir. Med.* 1982; 3:135-217.
3. Cohen, M. H.: Natural history of lung cancer. *Clin. Chest Med.* 1982; 3:229-241.
4. Ianuzzi, M. C., Scoggin, C. H. Small cell lung cancer.: *Am. Rev. Respir. Dis.* 1986; 134:593-608.

ALLERGIC ANGITIS AND GRANULOMATOSIS (CHURG-STRAUSS SYNDROME)

1. Leavitt , R. Y., Fauci, A. S.: Pulmonary vasculitis. *Am. Rev. Respir. Dis.* 1986; 134:149-166.
2. Fulmer, J. D., Kaltreider, H. B.: The pulmonary vasculitides. *Chest* 1982; 82:615-624.
3. Saldana, M. J.: Pulmonary vasculitides and related granulomatosis. *Semin. Respir. Med.* 1982; 4:113-122.

CYSTIC FIBROSIS

1. Fernard, G. W., Boat , T. F.: Cystic fibrosis: overview. *Semin. Roentgenol.* 1987; 22:87-96.
2. Davis, P. B (ed). Cystic fibrosis. *Semin. Respir. Med.* 1985; 6:243-333.
3. Davis, P. B., di Sant'Agnese, P. A.: Diagnosis and treatment of cystic fibrosis: an update. *Chest* 1984; 85:802-809.
4. Matthews, L. W., Drotar, D.: Cystic fibrosis-a challenging long-term chronic disease. *Pediatr. Clin. N. Am.* 1984; 31:133-152.

HISTOPLASMOSIS

1. Penn, R. L., Lambert, R. S., George, R. B.: Invasive fungal infections. The use of serologic tests in diagnosis and management. *Arch. Intern. Med.* 1983; 143:1215-1220.
2. Goodwin, R. A.Jr., Shapiro, J. L., Thurman, G. H., Thurman, S. S., Des Prez, R. M.: Disseminated histoplasmosis: clinical and pathologic correlations. *Medicine* (Baltimore) 1980; 59:1-33.
3. Ward, J. I., Weeks, M., Allen, D., Hutcheson, R. H. Jr., Anderson, R., Fraser, D. W., et. al.: Acute histoplasmosis: clinical, epidemiologic and serologic findings of an outbreak associated with exposure to a fallen tree. *Am. J. Med.* 1979; 66:587-595.
4. Goodwin, R. A. Jr., Des Prez, R. M.: Histoplasmosis. *Am. Rev. Respir. Dis.* 1978; 117:929-956.
5. Lowell, J. R., Shuford, E. H.: The value of the skin test and complement fixation test in the diagnosis of chronic pulmonary histoplasmosis. *Am. Rev. Respir. Dis.* 1976; 114:1069-1075.

IDIOPATHIC PULMONARY FIBROSIS (HAMMAN-RICH SYNDROME)

1. Turner-Warwick, M. (ed). Interstitial lung disease. *Semin. Respir. Med.* 1984;6:1-102.
2. Hamman, L., Rich, A. R.: Fulminating diffuse interstitial fibrosis of the lungs. *Trans. Am. Clin. Climatol. Assoc.* 1935; 51:154-163.

3. Crystal, R. G., Fulmer, J. D., Roberts, W. C., Moss, M. L., Line, B. R., Reynolds, H. Y.: Idiopathic pulmonary fibrosis. Clinical, histologic, radiographic, physiologic, scintigraphic, cytologic, and biochemical aspects. *Ann. Intern.Med.* 1976; 85:769-788.

IMMOTILE CILIA SYNDROME
1. Afzelius, B. A.: "Immotile-cilia" syndrome and ciliary abnormalities induced by infection and injury. *Am. Rev. Respir. Med.* 1981; 124:107-109.
2. Rossman, C. M., Forrest, J. B., Lee, R. M. K. W., Newhouse, M. T.: The dyskinetic cilia syndrome: ciliary motility in immotile cilia syndrome *Chest* 1980; 78:580-582.
3. Handelsman, D. J., Conway, A. J., Boylan, L. M., Turtle, J. R.: Young's syndrome. Obstructive azoospermia and chronic sinopulmonary infections. *N. E. J. M.* 1984; 310:3-9.

MESOTHELIOMA, PLEURAL
1. Legha, S. S., Muggia, F. M.: Pleural mesothelioma: clinical features and therapeutic implications. *Ann. Intern. Med.* 1977; 87:613-621.
2. Chahinian, A. P., Pajak, T. F., Holland, J. F., Norton, L., Ambinder, R. M., Mandel, E. M.: Diffuse malignant mesothelioma. Prospective evaluation of 69 patients. *Ann. Intern. Med.* 1982; 96:746-755.
3. Antman, K. H.: Malignant mesothelioma. *N. E. J. M.* 1980; 303:200-202.

PNEUMOCONIOSIS
1. Kleinerman, J., Merchant , J. A. Occupational lung diseases: silicosis, coalworkers' pneumoconiosis, amd miscellaneous pneumoconiosis.
   In Baum, G. L., Wolinsky, E. (eds): Textbook of Pulmonary Diseases 3rd Ed. Boston, Little, Brown, and Co. 1983, pp 743-768.
2. Kleinerman, J., Merchant , J. A. Occupational lung diseases: asbestosis-, talc-,and beryllium related respiratory diseases. In Baum, G. L., Wolinsky, E. (eds): Textbook of Pulmonary Diseases 3rd Ed. Boston, Little, Brown and Co. 1983, pp 769-788.

PNEUMONIA
1. Fick, R. B. Jr., Reynolds, H. Y.: Changing spectrum of pneumonia-news media creation or clinical reality? *Am. J. Med.* 1983; 74:1-8.
2. Davidson, M., Tempest , B., Palmer, D. L.: Bacteriologic diagnosis of acute pneumonia. Comparison of sputum, transtracheal aspirates, and lung aspirates. *J. A. M. A.* 1976; 235:158-163.

3. Toews, G. B.: Nosocomial pneumonia. *Clin. Chest Med.* 1987; 8:467-479.
4. Bartlett , J. G.: Anaerobic bacterial infections of the lung. *Chest* 1987; 91:901-909.

PNEUMOCYSTIS CARINII
1. Kovaks, J. A., Hiemenz, J. W., Macher, A. M., Stover, D., Murray, H. W., Shelhamer, J., et. al.: Pneumocystis carinii pneumonia: a comparison between patients with the acquired immunodeficiency syndrome and patients with other immunodeficiencies. *Ann. Intern. Med.* 1984; 100:663-671.
2. Macfarlane, J. T., Finch, R. G.: Pneumocystis carinii pneumonia. *Thorax* 1985; 40:561-570.
3. Mills, J.: Pneumocystis carinii and Toxoplasma gondii infections in patients with AIDS. *Rev. Infect. Dis.* 1986; 8:1001-1011.

PNEUMOTHORAX
1. Johnston, R. F., Green, R. A.: Pneumothorax. In Baum, G. L., Wolinsky, E. (eds): Textbook of Pulmonary Diseases, 3rd Ed. Boston, Little, Brown and Co. 1983, pp 1327-1341.
2. Fraser, R. G., Pare, J. A. Diagnosis of Diseases of the Chest, 2nd Ed. Philadelphia: W.B. Saunders Co. 1977, pp 594-601.
3. Felson, B.: Chest Roentgenology. Philadelphia: W.B. Saunders Co. 1973, pp 366-371.

PULMONARY EMBOLUS
1. Heim, C. R., Des Prez, R. M.: Pulmonary embolism; a review. *Adv. Intern. Med.* 1986; 31:187-212.
2. Hull, R. D., Hirsh, J., Carter, C. J. Jay, R. M., Dodd, P. E., Ockelford, P. A., et. al.: Pulmonary angiography, ventilation lung scanning, and venography for clinically suspected pulmonary embolism with abnormal perfusion lung scan. *Ann. Intern. Med.* 1983; 98:891-899.
3. Hull, R. D., Hirsh, J., Carter, C. J. Jay, R. M., Dodd, P. E., Ockelford, P. A., et. al.: Diagnostic efficacy of impedance plethysmography for clinically suspected deep-vein thrombosis. A randomized trial. *Ann. Intern. Med.* 1985; 102:21-28.
4. Fulkerson, W. J., Coleman, R. E., Ravin, C. E., Saltzman, H. A.: Diagnosis of pulmonary embolism. *Arch. Intern. Med.* 1986; 146:961-967.
5. West, J. W.: Pulmonary embolism. *Med. Clin. N. Am.* 1986; 70:877-894.

SARCOIDOSIS

1. Sharma, O. P.: Sarcoidosis: clinical, laboratory , and immunologic aspects. *Semin. Roentgenol.* 1985; 20:340-355.
2. Bascom, R., Johns, C. J.: The natural history and management of sarcoidosis. *Adv. Intern. Med.* 1986; 31:213-241.
3. Winterbauer, R. H., Belic, N., Moores, K. D.: A clinical interpretation of bilateral hilar adenopathy. *Ann. Intern. Med.* 1973;78:65-71.
4. Thrasher, D. R., Briggs, D. D. Jr.: Pulmonary sarcoidosis. *Clin. Chest Med.* 1982; 3:537-563.

TUBERCULOSIS

1. American Thoracic Society. Diagnostic standards and classification of tuberculosis and other mycobacterial diseases. *Am. Rev. Respir. Dis.* 1981; 123:343-351.
2. American Thoracic Society. The tuberculin skin test. *Am. Rev. Respir. Dis.* 1981; 124:356-363.
3. American Thoracic Society. Treatment of tuberculosis and tuberculosis infection in adults and children. *Am. Rev. Respir. Dis.* 1986; 134:355-363.
4. Khan, M. A., Kovnat, D. M., Bachus, B., Whitcomb, M. E., Brody, J. S., Snider, G. L.: Clinical and roentgenographic spectrum of pulmonary tuberculosis in the adult. *Am. J. Med.* 1977;62:31-38.

RHEUMATOLOGY

The number, types and priority of tests ordered must be individualized for each patient, consequently the tests listed for each disease in this chapter are not prioritized and are not exhaustive.

ANKYLOSING SPONDYLITIS
- BLOOD - May have increased WBC, ESR, and complement activity, mild anemia.
- CEREBRAL SPINAL FLUID - May have elevated protein.
- HISTOCOMPATIBILITY ANTIGEN STUDIES- HLA-B_{27} positive in >90% in whites, >50% in blacks.
- RADIOGRAPHY - Sacroiliitis, early ossification of vertebral ligaments and joints later in course of disease.

DERMATO/POLYMYOSITIS
- BLOOD - Usually elevated CPK, Aldolase, AST, LDH, ALT and ESR, in some cases Rheumatoid Factor and Antinuclear Antibodies are positive.
- URINE - Myoglobulinuria during acute illness may occur.
- BIOPSY - Muscle, shows myositis in two-thirds.
- EMG - Myopathic abnormalities.

GOUT
- BLOOD - Urate usually greater than or equal to 7.0 mg/dl in males and 6.0 mg/dl in females.
- Synovial Fluid - Negatively birefringent crystals usually seen in the neutrophils.
- GRAM STAIN - No organisms present.

HYPERSENSITIVITY VASCULITIS
- BLOOD - Usually mild leukocytosis with or without eosinophilia. Creatinine, CPK, Cryoglobulins, Rheumatoid Factor and ESR may be elevated .
- URINE - Proteinuria, and hematuria may be seen.
- BIOPSY - Skin shows leukocytoclastic vasculitis.

INFECTIOUS ARTHRITIS
- Synovial Fluid - Gram stain and culture are positive in the majority of non-gonococcal infections.
- BLOOD - Leukocytosis may be present.
- RADIOGRAPHY - Involved joint may be normal at first with osteopenia and erosions occurring later in the course.
- RADIOISOTOPIC SCAN - Shows increased uptake (helpful in localizing infection, particularly axial infection).

JUVENILE RHEUMATOID ARTHRITIS
- •BLOOD - Usually elevated ESR, microcytic hypochromic anemia. Elevated titer of Rheumatoid Factor in 10-20%, ANA present in 40%.
- •RADIOGRAPHY - Early: soft tissue swelling and juxta-articular demineralization.

KAWASAKI DISEASE (MUCOCUTANEOUS LYMPH NODE SYNDROME)
- •BLOOD - Mild anemia, leukocytosis with left shift, marked thrombocytosis, increased ESR, elevated IgE may be seen.
- •URINE - Pyuria, and proteinuria may be seen.
- •CEREBRAL SPINAL FLUID - May show pleocytosis with lymphocyte predominance.
- •2-D ECHOCARDIOGRAPHY - May show coronary aneurysm.
- •RADIOGRAPHY - CXR may show enlarged heart (secondary to pericarditis with effusion).

LYME DISEASE
- •BLOOD - Elevated anti-*Borellia burgdorferi* antibodies (IgM, IgG). Usually elevated total IgM, elevated AST.
- •Synovial Fluid Analysis - >2000 cells mostly PMNs.
- •Cerebral Spinal Fluid - Lymphocytes in those with meningitis.

OSTEOARTHRITIS
- •BLOOD - ANA negative, ESR normal, Rheumatoid Factor negative.
- •Synovial Fluid Analysis - Leukocyte count < 2000 /mm^3, mostly mononuclear cells.
- •RADIOGRAPHY - Initially normal, later osteophytes, eburnation and joint space narrowing.

POLYARTERITIS NODOSA
- •BLOOD - Usually shows leukocytosis with left shift, anemia, thrombocytosis, elevated globulins and ESR, 30% of patients are Hepatitis B surface antigen positive.
- •URINE - Proteinuria, and casts may be seen.
- •ANGIOGRAPHY- Usually, small aneurysms at the aortic bifurcation.
- •BIOPSY - Of affected tissue may show characteristic vasculitis, Non-involved tissue usually negative.

POLYMYALGIA RHEUMATICA
- BLOOD - Elevated ESR and hypochromic or normochromic anemia and serum protein abnormalities (variable types) may be seen.

PSEUDOGOUT
- Synovial Fluid Analysis - Large numbers of PMNs during acute attack, polarized light reveals positively birefringent crystals.
- RADIOGRAPHY - Chondrocalcinosis in involved joint may be seen.

PSORIATIC ARTHRITIS
- BLOOD - Hyperuricemia may be seen, negative rheumatoid factor.
- RADIOGRAPHY - Destruction of isolated joints, osteolysis, bony ankylosis, "pencil-in-cup" deformity most commonly found in distal interphalangeal joints. Lumbosacral spine may show sacroiliitis and ossification of the ligaments.

REITER'S SYNDROME
- BLOOD - Normochromic anemia, leukocytosis, elevated ESR may be seen.
- URINE - Microscopic hematuria and pyuria may be seen.
- SLIT LAMP - Iridocyclitis may be seen.
- RADIOGRAPHY - Affected joints may demonstrate juxta-articular osteoporosis, sacroiliitis, ankylosing spondylitis (syndesmophytes bridging the vertebrae).
- Synovial Fluid Analysis - Elevated PMN's.

RHEUMATIC FEVER
- BLOOD - Elevated ASO titer (Antistreptolysin O), streptozyme antibodies, and acute phase reactants and anemia may be seen.

RHEUMATOID ARTHRITIS
- BLOOD - Rheumatoid Factor positive, normochromic normocytic anemia, elevated ESR, ceruloplasmin and C-reactive protein, T4/T8 ratio increased, and thrombocytosis may be seen.
- RADIOGRAPHY - Juxta-articular osteoporosis, soft tissue swelling, joint space narrowing, bony erosions and cysts may be seen.
- Synovial Fluid Analysis - Leukocytosis with left shift, decreased glucose, fair to poor mucin clot are typical.

SCLERODERMA
- •BLOOD - Elevated ESR, mild anemia, rheumatoid factor positive, antinuclear antibodies, Anti-Scl-70 positive, centromere antinuclear antibodies (most common in the CREST syndrome) may be seen.
- •BIOPSY - Skin, esophagus, intestine or synovia typically show increased collagen formation

SJOGREN'S SYNDROME
- •BLOOD - Rheumatoid factor, anti-nuclear antibody, SSA and SSB autoantibody are often positive. Circulating immune complexes, leukopenia, elevated ESR, thrombocytosis and autoantibodies may be seen.
- •URINE - Sometimes renal tubular acidosis with decreased creatinine clearance and elevated pH.
- •BIOPSY - Minor salivary glands show lymphocytic infiltrate and acinar destruction.

SYSTEMIC LUPUS ERYTHEMATOSUS
- •BLOOD - Elevated ESR, anemia, leukopenia with decreased lymphocytes, low complement and decreased platelets are often seen. Antinuclear antibody in 95%, positive VDRL, Anti-Sm, and LE-cells may be seen.
- •URINE - Proteinuria, hematuria and casts may be found.
- •RADIOGRAPHY - CXR may show pleural and/or pericardial effusion. Joint films may demonstrate non-destructive arthritis.
- •EKG - May have evidence of pericarditis
  (See Nonbacterial Verrucous Endocarditis for further cardiac manifestations).

TAKAYASU'S ARTERITIS (AORTIC ARCH SYNDROME, PULSELESS DISEASE)
- •BLOOD - Usually elevated gamma globulins (mostly IgM), and ESR, mild anemia and leukocytosis.
- •ARTERIOGRAPHY/ANGIOGRAPHY- Segmental narrowing with post stenotic dilatation.

TEMPORAL (GIANT CELL) ARTERITIS
- BIOPSY - Temporal Artery (diagnostic study) shows giant cell arteritis, nonspecific white cell infiltration and intimal fibrosis with destruction of elastin.
- BLOOD - Typically ESR > 50, elevated WBC with left shift, moderate normocytic normochromic anemia, protein electrophoresis may show elevated gamma globulins. Rouleaux formation and immune complexes can occur. Liver function tests may be abnormal.
- Cerebral Spinal Fluid - May have elevated protein.

WEGENERS GRANULOMATOSIS
- BLOOD - Usually elevated ESR, acute phase reactants, anemia
- URINE - Hematuria, and proteinuria may be seen.
- RADIOGRAPHY - Sinusitis, lung infiltration may be seen.
- BIOPSY (Lung is the preferred site) - granulomatous vasculitis may be seen.

RHEUMATOLOGY REFERENCES

ANKYLOSING SPONDYLITIS
1. Gilliland, B. C. Ankylosing Spondylitis. In Harrison's Principles of Internal Medicine, 11th Ed. New York, McGraw Hill. 1987, pp 1434-1436.
2. Calin, A. Ankylosing Spondylitis. In Panayi, G. S. (ed). Philadelphia, W. B. Saunders. *Clin. Rheum. Dis.* 1985; 11:41-60.

DERMATO/POLYMYOSITIS
1. Bradley, W. G. Dermatomyositis and polymyositis In Harrison's Principles of Internal Medicine, 11th Ed. New York, McGraw Hill 1987, pp 2069-72.
2. Hochberg, M. C., Feldman, D., Stevens, M. B.: Adult onset polymyositis-dermatomyositis: an analysis of clinical and laboratory features and survival in 76 patients with a review of the literature. *Semin. Arthr. Rheum.* 1986; 15:168-178.

GOUT
1. Kelley, W. N. (ed), et. al. Textbook of Rheumatology, 2nd Ed. Philadelphia, W. B. Saunders Co. 1985, pp 1359-1381.
2. Evans, T. Gout and Pseudogout. In Barnes, H. V. (ed): Clinical Medicine: Selected Problems with Pathophysiologic Correlations, 1st Ed. Chicago, Year Book Medical Publishers 1988, pp 838-844.

HYPERSENSITIVITY VASCULITIS
1. Faryna, A. Systemic Vasculitis. In Barnes, H. V. (ed): Clinical Medicine: Selected Problems with Pathophysiologic Correlations, 1st Ed. Chicago, Year Book Medical Publishers 1988, pp 807-815.

INFECTIOUS ARTHRITIS
1. Goldenberg, D. L., Reed, J. I.: Bacterial Arthritis. *N. E. J. M.* 1985; 312:764-771.
2. Faryna, A., Goldenberg, K. Septic Arthritis. In Barnes, H. V. (ed): Clinical Medicine, 1st Ed. Chicago, Year Book Medical Publishers 1988, pp 844-849.

JUVENILE ARTHRITIS
1. Calabro, J. J. Juvenile Arthritis. In McCarty, D. J. (ed): Arthritis and Allied Conditions - A textbook of Rheumatology, 10th Ed. Philadelphia, Lea and Febiger 1985, pp 799-810.

2. Levinson, J. E., Balz, G. P, Hess, E. V.: Report of studies on Juvenile Arthritis. *Arth. Rheum.* 1977; 20:189-190.

KAWASAKI DISEASE (MUCOCUTANEOUS LYMPH NODE SYNDROME)
1. Conn, D. L, Hunder, G. G. Necrotizing Vasculitis. In Kelley, W. N. (ed): Textbook of Rheumatology, 2nd Ed. Philadelphia, W.B. Saunders Co. 1985, pp 1161.

LYME DISEASE
1. Steere, A. C., Schoen, R. T., Taylor, E.: The clinical evolution of Lyme Arthritis. *Ann. Intern. Med.* 1987;107:725-731.

OSTEOARTHRITIS
1. Gilliland, B. C. Degenerative joint disease. In Harrison's Principles of Internal Medicine, 11th Ed. New York, McGraw Hill 1987, pp.1456-1458.

POLYARTERITIS NODOSA
1. Faryna, A. Systemic Vasculitis. In Barnes, H. V. (ed) : Clinical Medicine: Selected Problems with Pathophysiologic Correlations, 1st Ed. Chicago, Year Book Medical Publishers 1988, pp 807-815.

POLYMYALGIA RHEUMATICA
1. Paty, J. G. Polymyalgia Rheumatica. In Barnes, H. V. (ed) : Clinical Medicine, 1st Ed. Chicago, Year Book Medical Publishers 1988, pp 824-827.

PSEUDOGOUT
1. Evans, T. Gout and Pseudogout. In Barnes, H. V. (ed): Clinical Medicine: Selected Problems with Pathophysiologic Correlations, 1st Ed. Chicago, Year Book Medical Publishers 1988, pp 838-844.

PSORIATIC ARTHRITIS
1. Laurent , M. R. Psoriatic Arthritis. In Panayi, G. S. (ed): Clin. Rheum. Dis. Philadelphia, W. B. Saunders. 1985;11:61-85.

REITERS SYNDROME
1. Mountsopoulus, H. M. Reiter's Syndrome and Behcet's Syndrome. In Harrison's Principles of Internal Medicine, 11th Ed. New York, McGraw Hill 1987, pp 1436-1437.
2. Primer in Rheumatic Diseases, 8th Ed. Am Rheum Assoc. 1983, pp 88-91.

RHEUMATIC FEVER
1. Bisno, A. L. Rheumatic Fever. In Mandell, G. L.(ed) Principles and Practice of Infectious Disease, 2nd Ed. New York, J. Wiley & Sons. 1985, pp 1133-1137.
2. Stollerman, G. H. Rheumatic Fever. In Harrison's Principles of Internal Medicine, 11th Ed. New York, McGraw Hill 1987, pp 951-956.

RHEUMATOID ARTHRITIS
1. Lipsky, P. E. Rheumatoid Arthritis. In Harrison's Principles of Internal Medicine, 11th Ed. New York, McGraw Hill 1987, pp 1423-1428.
2. Faryna, A. Rheumatoid Arthritis. In Barnes, H. V. (ed) et al: Clinical Medicine, 1st Ed. Chicago, Year Book Medical Publishers. 1988, pp 793-798.

SCLERODERMA
1. Primer in Rheumatic Disease, 8th Ed. Am Rheum Assoc. 1983, pp 59-65.
2. Gilliland, B. C. Progressive Systemic Sclerosis. In Harrison's Principles of Internal Medicine, 11th Ed. New York, McGraw Hill 1987, pp 1428-1432.

SJOGREN'S SYNDROME
1. Primer in Rheumatic Disease, 8th Ed. Am Rheum Assoc. 1983, pp 77-79.
2. Lane, H. C., Fauci, A. S. Sjogren's Syndrome. In Harrison's Principles of Internal Medicine, 11th Ed. New York, McGraw Hill 1987, pp 1433-1434.

SYSTEMIC LUPUS ERYTHEMATOSUS
1. Hahn, B. H. Systemic Lupus Erythematosus. In Harrison's Principles of Internal Medicine, 11th Ed. New York, McGraw Hill 1987, pp 1418-1427.
2. Hawkins, R. A. Systemic Lupus Erythematosus. In Barnes, H. V. (ed) et al: Clinical Medicine: Selected Problems with Pathophysiologic Correlations, 1st Ed. Chicago, Year Book Medical Publishers 1988, pp 799-807.

TAKAYASU'S ARTERITIS (AORTIC ARCH SYNDROME, PULSELESS DISEASE)
1. Primer in Rheumatic Disease, 8th Ed. Am Rheum Assoc. 1983, pp 74.

2. Fauci, A. S. The vasculitic syndromes. In Harrison's Principles of Internal Medicine, 11th Ed. New York, McGraw Hill 1987, pp 1444.

TEMPORAL ARTERITIS
1. Fauci, A. S. The vasculitic syndromes. In Harrison's Principles of Internal Medicine, 11th Ed. New York, McGraw Hill 1987, pp 1443.
2. Huston, K. A., Hunder, G. G., Lie, J. T., Kennedy, R. H., Elveback, L. R.: Temporal Arteritis: A 25-year epidemiologic, clinical and pathologic study. *Ann. Intern. Med.* 1978;88:162-167.

WEGENERS GRANULOMATOSIS
1. Fauci, A. S. The vasculitic syndromes. In Harrison's Principles of Internal Medicine, 11th Ed. New York, McGraw Hill 1987, pp 1442-1443.

SECTION IV

Test Characteristics and Predictive Value

Mark M. Redding, M.D.
Elliott J. Fegelman, M.D.
Robert H. Edwards, M.D.
Sarah A. Redding, M.D.
Richard D. Wetmore, M.D.
Anthony W. Clarke, M.D.
Wallace M. Combs, M.D.
Curtis B. Everson, M.D.
Kevin L. Riddle, M.D.
Patricia J. Rubin, M.D.

The following data were derived from the references provided at the end of this section. This information may be applicable to your clinical situation assuming that your laboratory has operating characteristics similar to those used in our references.

NOMOGRAM

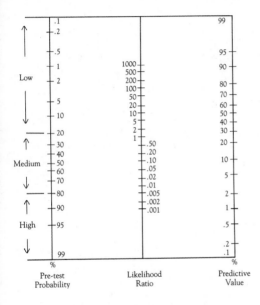

Figure 1. Nomogram for determining predictive value of a diagnostic test using the likelihood ratio. To use the nomogram, find the Pre-test Probability on the left hand scale and the Likelihood Ratio on the center scale. Draw a straight line connecting these two points and extend the line to intercept the Predictive Value on the right hand scale (modified from Fagan T.J.: *N. Engl. J. Med.* 1975;293:257. Reproduced by permission).

	SENS	SPEC	LR +	LR -
ACID PHOSPHATASE				
Prostatic Cancer				
Stage A	18	92	2.3	0.9
Stage B	33	92	4.1	0.7
Stage C	60	92	7.5	0.4
Stage D	91	92	11.4	0.1
BPH with infarction (transient)	100	92	12.5	<.1
ALANINE AMINO				
TRANSFERASE (ALT, SGPT)				
Alcoholic Hepatic Disease	75	87-95*	5.8-15.0	0.3
Biliary Inflammation	77	87-95*	5.8-15.4	0.2
Cancer of Bile Duct	95*	87-95*	7.3-19.0	0.1
Cholelithiasis	89	87-95*	6.8-17.8	0.1
Cholestasis, "Mild"	26	87-95*	2.0-5.2	0.8-0.9
Cholestasis, "Severe"	77	87-95*	5.9-15.4	0.3
Cirrhosis, Portal	45-64	87-95*	3.5-12.8	0.4-0.6
Cirrhosis, Primary Biliary	96*	87-95*	7.4-19.2	<.1
Hepatic Metastasis	74	87-95*	5.7-14.8	0.3
Hepatitis, Chronic Active	85	87-95*	6.5-17.0	0.2
Hepatitis, Infectious, "early"	100	87-95*	7.7-20.0	<.1
Hepatitis, Infectious, "late"	100	87-95*	7.7-20.0	<.1
Pancreatic Cancer, (Head)	100	87-95*	7.7-20.0	<.1
ALDOSTERONE,				
NONSUPPRESSIBLE*				
(concentration)				
Primary Aldosteronism*	72*	91*	8.0	0.3
ALDOSTERONE,				
NONSUPPRESSIBLE*				
(excretion rate)				
Primary Aldosteronism*	96*	93*	13.7	<.1
ALKALINE PHOSPHATASE				
Alcoholic Hepatic Disease	48	92	6.0	0.6
Biliary Inflammation	85	92	10.6	0.2
Cancer of Bile Duct	100*	92	12.5	<.1
Cardiovascular Disease	37	92	4.6	0.7
Cholelithiasis	97	92	12.1	<.1

LR+ = Likelihood ratio of a Positive Test.
LR - = Likelihood ratio of a Negative Test.
* See reference notes for accurate interpretation.

(Cont.)	SENS	SPEC	LR +	LR -
Cirrhosis, Portal	67*	92	8.4	0.4
Cirrhosis, Primary Biliary	100*	92	12.5	<.1
Diabetes Mellitus, "uncontrolled"	50	92	6.3	0.5
Hepatic Metastasis (all sources)	85	92	10.6	0.2
Colorectal Cancer	64*	82*	3.6	0.4
Hepatitis, Chronic Active	74	92	9.3	0.3
Hepatitis, Infectious, "early"	94	92	11.8	0.1
Hepatitis, Infectious, "late"	82	92	10.3	0.2
Intrahepatic Cholestasis	79*	92	9.9	0.2
Pancreatic Cancer, (Head)	100	92	12.5	<.1

ALPHA-FETOPROTEIN	SENS	SPEC	LR +	LR -
Hepatitis: Chronic Active, Drug and Viral	25-36	>99	25.0-36.0	0.6-0.8
Hepatomas	72	>99	72	0.3
Pancreatic Cancer	23	>99	23	0.8
Testicular Teratocarcinoma	75	>99	75	0.3
Yolk Sac Neoplasms	100	>99	100	<.1

AMMONIA*	SENS	SPEC	LR +	LR -
Hepatic Insufficiency*				
without Cerebral Dysfunction	67*	>99	67	0.3
with Cerebral Dysfunction	75*	>99	75	0.3
with Hepatic Coma	100*	>99	100	<.1
Reye's Syndrome*	80	>99	80	0.2

AMYLASE	SENS	SPEC	LR +	LR -
Abdominal Procedure	35	71-89*	1.2-3.2	0.7-0.9
Appendicitis, Acute	5	71-89*	0.2-0.5	1.1-1.3
Cholecystitis, Acute	22	71-89*	0.8-2.0	0.9-1.1
Pancreatitis, Acute	95	71-89*	3.3-8.6	0.1
Mumps	85	71-89*	2.9-7.7	0.2
Perforated Ulcer	30	71-89*	1.0-2.7	0.8-1.0

ANTI-NUCLEAR ANTIBODY	SENS	SPEC	LR +	LR -
CREST Syndrome	70-90	69-95	2.3-18.0	0.1-0.4
Dermatomyositis/Polymyositis	49-74	69-95	1.6-14.8	0.3-0.7

LR+ = Likelihood ratio of a Positive Test.
LR - = Likelihood ratio of a Negative Test.
* See reference notes for accurate interpretation.

	SENS	SPEC	LR +	LR -
(Cont.)				
Drug Induced Lupus	95-100	69-95	3.1-20.0	<.1-0.1
Mixed Connective Tissue Disease	95-100	69-95	3.1-20.0	<.1-0.1
Rheumatoid Arthritis	40-60	69-95	1.0-1.9	0.6-1.0
Systemic Sclerosis	60-90	69-95	1.9-18.0	0.1-0.4
Sjogren's Syndrome	75-90	69-95	2.4-18.0	0.1-0.2
Systemic Lupus Erythematosus	95-100	69-95*	3.1-20.0	<.1-0.1
ANTI-RIBONUCLEAR PROTEIN				
Mixed Connective Tissue Disease	95-100	>99	95-100	<.1
Systemic Lupus Erythematosus	30-40	>99	30-40	0.6-0.7
ANTI-SM ANTIBODY				
Mixed Connective Tissue Disease	8	>99	8.0	0.9
Systemic Lupus Erythematosus	30-40	>99	30-40	0.6
ANTITHROMBIN III				
Decreased Activity				
Disseminated Intravascular Coagulation	74-79	>95	14.8-15.8	0.2-0.3
Liver Disease	84	>95	16.0	0.2
Post Operative	88	>95	17.6	0.1
Preeclampsia	76	91	8.4	0.3
ASPARTATE AMINOTRANSFERASE (AST, SGOT)				
Alcoholic Hepatic Disease	78	87-99*	6.0-78.0	0.2-0.3
Biliary Inflammation	73	87-99*	5.6-73.0	0.3
Cancer of Bile Duct	100*	87-99*	7.7-100	<.1
Cholelithiasis	95	87-99*	7.3-95	0.1
Cholestasis, "Mild"	28	87-99*	2.2-28	0.7-0.8

LR+ = Likelihood ratio of a Positive Test.
LR - = Likelihood ratio of a Negative Test.
* See reference notes for accurate interpretation.

	SENS	SPEC	LR +	LR -
(Cont.)				
Cholestasis, "Severe"	88	87-99*	6.8-88	0.1
Cirrhosis, Portal	81-90	87-99*	6.2-90.0	0.1-0.2
Cirrhosis, Primary Biliary	100*	87-99*	7.7-100	<.1
Hepatic Metastasis	86	87-99*	6.6-86.0	0.1-0.2
Hepatitis, Chronic Active	87	87-99*	6.7-87.0	0.1
Hepatitis, Infectious , "Early"	100	87-99*	7.7-100	<.1
Hepatitis, Infectious, "Late"	93	87-99*	7.2-93.0	0.1
Myocardial Infarction	53	82-99*	2.9-53.0	0.5-0.6
Pancreatic Cancer, (Head)	100	87-99*	7.7-100	<.1

ASPARTATE AMINOTRANS- FERASE, Serial Tests				
Myocardial Infarction	95-97	86-90	6.8-9.7	<.1-0.1

B_{12}				
Megaloblastic Anemia*	<18	99	18.0	0.8

BILE ACIDS (Fasting)				
Cholestasis, "Mild"	93	88-99*	7.8-93.0	0.1
Cholestasis, "Severe"	98	88-99*	8.2-98.0	<.1
Cirrhosis	93	88-99*	7.8-93.0	0.1
Hepatitis, Acute	97	88-99*	9.1-97.0	<.1

BILIRUBIN, TOTAL				
Cholestasis, "Mild"	26	87-98	2.0-13.0	0.8-0.9
Cholestasis, "Severe"	68	87-98	5.2-34.0	0.3-0.4
Cirrhosis	65	87-98	5.0-32.5	0.4
Hepatitis, Acute	93	87-98	7.2-46.5	0.1

BLEEDING TIME				
von Willebrand's Disease	72	>99	72	0.3
Thrombocytopathy	43	>99	43	0.6

C-PEPTIDE				
Diabetes Mellitus, Type I	94	80*	4.7	0.1

LR+ = Likelihood ratio of a Positive Test.
LR - = Likelihood ratio of a Negative Test.
* See reference notes for accurate interpretation.

	SENS	SPEC	LR +	LR -
C-PEPTIDE Glucagon StimulationTEST				
Diabetes Mellitus, Type I	94	96*	23.5	0.1
C-REACTIVE PROTEIN				
Epiglottitis (Children)	100	88-99	8.3-100	<.1
Meningitis, Bacterial (Children)	95	99	95	0.1
Pharyngitis, Acute Streptococcal (Children)	78	47-99*	1.5-78	0.2-0.5
Rheumatoid Arthritis Severity Score:*				
1 (mild)	40*	99	40	0.6
2	73	99	73	0.3
3	94	99	94	0.1
4 (severe)	100*	99	100	<.1
CALCIUM				
Hyperparathyroidism	89	94	14.8	0.1
cAMP, URINE				
Primary Hypoparathyroidism	89	95	17.8	0.1
CARCINOEMBRYONIC ANTIGEN (CEA)				
Alcoholism	65	70-80	2.2-3.3	0.4-0.5
Breast Cancer	47-66	70-80	1.6-3.3	0.4-0.8
Colon Cancer				
Duke's Stage A	58	70-80	1.9-2.9	0.5-0.6
Duke's Stage B	68	70-80	2.3-3.4	0.4-0.5
Duke's Stage C	71	70-80	2.4-3.6	0.4
Duke's Stage D	81	70-80	2.7-4.1	0.2-0.3
Emphysema	57	70-80	1.9-2.9	0.5-0.6
Gastric Cancer	46-61	70-80	1.5-3.1	0.5-0.8
Hyperplasia	21	70-80	0.7-1.1	1.0-1.1
Ileitis	40	70-80	1.3-2.0	0.8-0.9
Lung Cancer	74	70-80	2.5-3.7	0.3-0.4
Pancreatic Cancer	77-91	70-80	2.6-4.6	0.1-0.3

LR+ = Likelihood ratio of a Positive Test.
LR - = Likelihood ratio of a Negative Test.
* See reference notes for accurate interpretation.

	SENS	SPEC	LR +	LR -
(Cont.)				
Pancreatitis	53	70-80	1.8-2.7	0.6-0.7
Pneumonia	46	70-80	1.5-2.3	0.7-0.8
Prostatic Cancer	44	70-80	1.5-2.2	0.7-0.8
Transplants	56	70-80	1.9-2.8	0.6
Ulcerative Colitis	31	70-80	1.0-1.6	0.9-1.0

CAROTENE				
Decreased, Malabsorption	95	77-88	4.1-7.9	0.1

CATECHOLAMINES				
Pheochromocytoma	94-100	97*	31.3-33.3	<.1-0.1

CENTROMERE / KINETOCHORE				
CREST Syndrome	70-90	>95	14.0-18.0	0.1-0.3
Dermatomyositis/Polymyositis..	< 5	>95	1.0	1.0
Drug Induced Lupus	< 5	>95	1.0	1.0
Mixed Connective Tissue Disease	< 5	>95	1.0	1.0
Systemic Lupus Erythematosus	<5	>95	1.0	1.0
Systemic Sclerosis	30	>95	6.0	0.7
Sjogren's Syndrome	<5	>95	1.0	1.0

CERULOPLASMIN				
Decreased Wilson's Disease: Symptomatic and Asymptomatic	98	>98	49.0	<.1

COPPER				
Decreased Wilson's Disease: Asymptomatic	77	>98	38.5	0.2

LR+ = Likelihood ratio of a Positive Test.
LR - = Likelihood ratio of a Negative Test.
* See reference notes for accurate interpretation.

	SENS	SPEC	LR +	LR -
COPPER, Urine				
Wilson's Disease:				
Asymptomatic	80	>98	40.0	0.2
Symptomatic	>99	>98	49.5	<.1
CORTISOL, 24 hr. URINE FREE (UFC)				
Cushing's Syndrome	94	91 - >99*	10.4-94.0	0.1
CORTISOL				
Cushing's 8 a.m.	40	71	1.4	0.8
Cushing's 4-9 p.m.	83	67	2.5	0.3
Cushing's midnight	96	96	24.0	<.1
CREATINE PHOSPHOKINASE MB FRACTION, Single Test				
Acute Myocardial Infarction*				
2-4 hours post onset of symptoms	26	88*	2.2	0.8
4-6 hours post onset of symptoms	75	88*	6.3	0.3
6-8 hours post onset of symptoms	95	88*	7.9	0.1
10-20 hours post onset of symptoms	100	88*	8.3	<.1
CREATINE PHOSPHOKINASE MB FRACTION, Serial Tests*				
Myocardial Infarction	93-100	99	93-100	<.1-0.1
CREATINE PHOSPHOKINASE, Total, Single Test				
Myocardial Infarction	38	80	1.9	0.8
CREATINE PHOSPHOKINASE, Total, Serial Tests				
Myocardial Infarction	95-98	67-78	2.9-4.5	<.1-0.1

LR+ = Likelihood ratio of a Positive Test.
LR - = Likelihood ratio of a Negative Test.
* See reference notes for accurate interpretation.

	SENS	SPEC	LR +	LR -
DEXAMETHASONE HIGH DOSE (2 mg) SUPPRESSION - TWO DAY				
Cushing's (17-OHCS, Urine)..	75	86	5.4	0.3
Cushing's (Cortisol)..................	79	>99	79	0.2

	SENS	SPEC	LR +	LR -
DEXAMETHASONE SUPPRESSION-OVERNIGHT LOW DOSE (1 mg)				
Cushing's	98	82	5.4	<.1
HIGH DOSE (8 mg)				
Cushing's	92	99	92	<.1

	SENS	SPEC	LR +	LR -
DNA, Double Stranded				
CREST...	<5	>95	1.0	1.0
Dermatomyositis/Polymyositis..	< 5	>95	1.0	1.0
Drug Induced Lupus	< 5	>95	1.0	1.0
Mixed Connective Tissue				
Disease.......................................	< 5	>95	1.0	1.0
Sjogren's Syndrome..................	<5	>95	1.0	1.0
Systemic Lupus				
Erythematosus...........................	50-70	>95	10.0-14.0	0.3-0.5
Systemic Sclerosis....................	<5	>95	1.0	1.0

	SENS	SPEC	LR +	LR -
DNA, Single Stranded				
Dermatomyositis/Polymyositis..	10-20	>80	0.5-1.0	1.0-1.1
Drug Induced Lupus	< 5	>80	0.3	1.2
Hepatitis, Chronic Active	60	>80	3.0	0.5
Mixed Connective Tissue				
Disease.......................................	10-20	>80	0.5-1.0	1.0-1.1
Mononucleosis...........................	40	>80	2.0	0.8
Myasthenia Gravis.....................	20	>80	1.0	1.0
Rheumatoid Arthritis...................	50-60	>80	2.5-3.0	0.5-0.6
Systemic Lupus				
Erythematosus...........................	60-70	>80	3.0-3.5	0.4-0.5
Systemic Sclerosis....................	10-20	>80	0.5-1.0	1.0-1.1
Sjogren's Syndrome..................	10-20	>80	0.5-1.0	1.0-1.1

LR+ = Likelihood ratio of a Positive Test.
LR - = Likelihood ratio of a Negative Test.
* See reference notes for accurate interpretation.

	SENS	SPEC	LR +	LR -
ERYTHROCYTE PROTOPORPHYRIN (Epp) Iron Deficiency Anemia *	61-74	96 - >99	15.3-74.0	0.3-0.4
FECAL FAT - QUALITATIVE Steatorrhea (Using Oil Red O or Sudan III)	72-100	96	18.1-25.0	<.1-0.3
FERRITIN Hemochromatosis (age <35 yrs)............................... Iron Deficiency Anemia*............	85 66-83	95 61-75	17.0 1.7-3.3	0.2 0.2-0.6
FIBRINOGEN/FIBRIN (FRAGMENT E) "Recent" Deep Vein Thrombosis..............................	99	65-84*	2.8-6.2	<.1
FOLIC ACID Macrocytic Anemia .... Anemia (of all types)...................	<18 2	99* 99*	18.0 2.0	0.8 1.0
FSH Gonadal Dysgenesis...................	100	95	20.0	<.1
FTA-AB Syphilis * Primary....................................... Secondary.................................. Early Latent (< 1 to 2 years) ... Late Latent (> 2 years).............	86-100 99 100 95	77 - >99 77 - >99 77 - >99 77 - >99	3.7-100 4.3-99.0 4.3-100 4.1-95.0	<.1-0.2 <.1 <.1 0.1
GAMMA-GLUTAMYL TRANSPEPTIDASE Alcohol Abuse Screen.............. Congestive Heart Failure .... Hepatic Metastasis .... Liver Disease*...........................	70 70 91 83*	82 82 82 82	3.9 3.9 5.1 4.6	0.4 0.4 0.1 0.2

LR+ = Likelihood ratio of a Positive Test.
LR - = Likelihood ratio of a Negative Test.
* See reference notes for accurate interpretation.

	SENS	SPEC	LR +	LR -
GROWTH HORMONE **(1 Hour Post Oral** **Glucose Load)** Acromegaly	100*	>99*	100	<.1
GROWTH HORMONE **(2 Hour Glucagon** **Stimulation Test)** Growth Hormone Deficiency	91	97	30.3	0.1
GROWTH HORMONE **(FASTING)** Acromegaly	71*	88*	5.9	0.3
HAPTOGLOBIN Decreased Hemolytic Disorders See Differential Section	83*	96*	20.8	0.2
HEMOGLOBIN A1C Diabetes Mellitus Gestational Diabetes	60* 63	91* 81	6.7 3.3	0.4 0.5
HEPATITIS A IgM Anti-HAV Acute Hepatitis A	100	99	100	<.1
HEPATITIS A TOTAL **Anti-HAV** Acute Hepatitis A	100	84	6.3	<.1
HEPATITIS B Anti-HBc Acute/Chronic HBV infection RIA EIA (Abbott) EIA (Organon)	99 100 90	92 95 89	12.4 20.0 8.2	<.1 <.1 0.1

LR+ = Likelihood ratio of a Positive Test.
LR - = Likelihood ratio of a Negative Test.
* See reference notes for accurate interpretation.

	SENS	SPEC	LR +	LR -
HEPATITIS B Anti-HBe				
Chronic carrier				
EIA (Abbott)............................	100	>99	100	<.1
EIA (Organon)........................	100	>99	100	<.1
HEPATITIS B Anti-HBs				
Seroconversion/Immunization				
RIA	96	99	96.0	<.1
EIA (Abbott)............................	100	>99	>99	<.1
EIA (Organon)........................	100	73	3.7	<.1
HEPATITIS B HBeAg				
Acute/Chronic HBV infection				
EIA (Abbott)............................	100	>99	100	<.1
EIA (Organon)........................	81	>99	81.0	0.2
HEPATITIS B HBsAg				
Early/late HBV infection				
RIA	93	99	93.0	0.1
RIA 30'.....................................	77	95	15.4	0.2
ELISA.......................................	75	98	37.5	0.3
RPHA..	49	99	49.0	0.5
LATEX......................................	31	94	5.2	0.7
Chronic HBV infection				
RIA	100	99	100	<.1
RIA 30'.....................................	100	95	20.0	<.1
ELISA.......................................	99.5	98	49.8	<.1
RPHA..	98	99	98.0	<.1
LATEX......................................	84	94	14.0	0.2
HETEROPHILE				
Horse Cell Agglutinin Test*				
Infectious Mononucleosis........	86-100*	93	12.3-14.3	<.1-0.2
Beef Hemolysis Test				
Infectious Mononucleosis........	69-100*	96 - >99	17.3-100	<.1-0.3
Sheep Cell Agglutinin Test*				
Infectious Mononucleosis........	69-80*	88	5.8-6.7	0.2-0.4

LR+ = Likelihood ratio of a Positive Test.
LR - = Likelihood ratio of a Negative Test.
* See reference notes for accurate interpretation.

	SENS	SPEC	LR +	LR -
HISTONES				
CREST Syndrome	<5	>95	1.0	1.0
Dermatomyositis/Polymyositis..	< 5	>95	1.0	1.0
Drug Induced Lupus	>95	>95	19.0	0.1
Mixed Connective Tissue Disease	< 5	>95	1.0	1.0
Rheumatoid Arthritis	15-20	>95	3.0-4.0	0.8-0.9
Sjogren's Syndrome	<5	>95	1.0	1.0
Systemic Lupus Erythematosus	70	>95	14.0	0.3
Systemic Sclerosis	<5	>95	1.0	1.0
HLA-B27				
Ankylosing Spondylitis (Whites)	92	92	11.5	0.1
Ankylosing Spondylitis (Blacks)	50	98	25.0	0.5
Reiter's Syndrome (Whites)	72	92	9.0	0.3
Reiter's Syndrome (Blacks)	40	98	20.0	0.6
HOMOVANILIC ACID (HVA), 24 HOUR URINE				
Neuroblastoma*	90	>99	90.0	0.1
Pheochromocytoma*	75	>99	75.0	0.3
HUMAN CHORIONIC GONADOTROPIN BETA SUBUNIT (BETA-HCG SERUM)				
Breast Cancer	12-21	>99	12.0-21.0	0.5-0.9
Choriocarcinoma	100	>99	100	<.1
Colorectal Cancer	12	>99	12.0	0.9
Embryonal Carcinoma	56	>99	56.0	0.4
Endometrial Cancer*	24	>99	24.0	0.8
Gastric Cancer	24	>99	24.0	0.8
Liver Neoplasm*	21	>99	21.0	0.8
Melanomas	10	>99	10.0	0.9
Ovarian Adenocarcinoma*	18-40	>99	18.0-40.0	0.6-0.8
Pancreatic Neoplasm*	33	>99	33.0	0.7
Pregnancy, Ectopic	100*	83*-99	5.9-100	<.1
Pregnancy, Intrauterine	99	>99	99.0	<.1

LR+ = Likelihood ratio of a Positive Test.
LR - = Likelihood ratio of a Negative Test.
* See reference notes for accurate interpretation.

(Cont.)	SENS	SPEC	LR +	LR -
Seminoma..................................	38*	>99	38.0	0.6
Uterine Cervical Cancer*	31	>99	31.0	0.7
Vulvar Cancer*..........................	33*	>99	33.0	0.7

HUMAN CHORIONIC GONADOTROPIN BETA SUBUNIT (BETA-HCG URINE)				
Pregnancy, Ectopic....................	60*	99	60	0.4
Pregnancy, Intrauterine	98	99	98.0	<.1

HUMAN IMMUNODEFICIENCY VIRUS (HIV) TESTS				
ELISA.......................................	68-86	74 - >99	2.6-86	0.1-0.4
Western Blot..............................	86-100	80 - >99	4.3-100	<.1-0.2

17-HYDROXYCORTICO-STEROID 24 HOUR URINE				
Cushing's Syndrome/Disease .	89	73-99*	3.3-89.0	0.1-0.2

5-HYDROXYINDOLACETIC ACID (5-HIAA) URINE				
Carcinoid....................................	73	>99	73	0.3

17-HYDROXYPROGESTRONE				
21-Hydroxylase Deficiency (CAH)	100*	>99	100	<.1

INSULIN ANTIBODIES (ELISA) Diabetes Mellitus				
With Insulin Treatment	100	>99*	100	<.1

IRON Hemochromatosis				
(age <35 yrs).............................	68	83	4.0	0.4
Iron Deficiency Anemia *	62-74	83 - >99	3.6-74	0.3-0.5

ISOAMYLASE				
Pancreatitis, Acute......................	92	85* - >95	6.1-18.4	0.1

LR+ = Likelihood ratio of a Positive Test.
LR - = Likelihood ratio of a Negative Test.
* See reference notes for accurate interpretation.

	SENS	SPEC	LR +	LR -
JO, NUCLEAR PROTEIN ANTIGEN				
CREST Syndrome..................	<5	>95	1.0	1.0
Dermatomyositis.................	5	>95	1.0	1.0
Drug Induced Lupus	< 5	>95	1.0	1.0
Mixed Connective Tissue Disease................................	< 5	>95	1.0	1.0
Polymyositis......................	31	>95	6.2	0.7
Sjogren's Syndrome...............	<5	>95	1.0	1.0
Systemic Sclerosis...............	<5	>95	1.0	1.0
Systemic Lupus Erythematosus	<5	>95	1.0	1.0

	SENS	SPEC	LR +	LR -
17-KETOSTEROIDS 24 HOUR URINE				
Cushing's Syndrome	65	83	3.8	0.4

	SENS	SPEC	LR +	LR -
LACTATE DEHYDROGENASE, Serial tests				
Acute Myocardial Infarction	95-98	72-94	3.4-16.3	<.1-0.1

	SENS	SPEC	LR +	LR -
LACTATE DEHYDROGENASE, Single test				
Acute Myocardial Infarction......	60	66	1.8	0.6

	SENS	SPEC	LR +	LR -
LDH ISOENZYMES				
Acute Myocardial Infarction LDH1 > LDH2	90-96	95-97	18.0-32.0	<.1-0.1

	SENS	SPEC	LR +	LR -
LIPASE				
Acute Pancreatitis......................	86.5	99	86.5	0.1

	SENS	SPEC	LR +	LR -
LUTEINIZING HORMONE				
Gonadal Dysgenesis.................	100*	>90*	100	<.1
Polycystic Ovary Disease..........	77*	>90*	7.7	0.3

	SENS	SPEC	LR +	LR -
MEAN CORPUSCULAR HEMOGLOBIN (MCH)				
Iron Deficiency Anemia *..........	97-100	83 ->99	5.7-100	<.1

LR+ = Likelihood ratio of a Positive Test.
LR - = Likelihood ratio of a Negative Test.
* See reference notes for accurate interpretation.

	SENS	SPEC	LR +	LR -
MEAN CORPUSCULAR VOLUME (MCV)				
Iron Deficiency Anemia *	85-100	83 - >99	5.0-100	<.1-0.6

	SENS	SPEC	LR +	LR -
METANEPHRINES (URINE)				
Pheochromocytoma	95-100	>95*	19.0-20.0	<.1-0.1

MONOSPOT (See Heterophile Antibody)

	SENS	SPEC	LR +	LR -
5-NUCLEOTIDASE				
Bile Duct Cancer	100*	88	8.3	<.1
Cardiovascular Disease	37	88	3.1	0.7
Cholelithiasis	94	88	7.8	0.1
Cirrhosis	71	88	5.9	0.3
Cirrhosis, Primary Biliary	100*	88	8.3	<.1
Hepatic Metastasis from				
Colorectal Cancer	52*	82*	2.9	0.6
Hepatitis, Chronic Active	74	88	6.2	0.3
Hepatitis, Infectious, "early"	100	88	8.3	<.1
Hepatitis, Infectious, "late"	68	88	5.7	0.4
Intrahepatic Cholestasis	66*	88	5.5	0.4
Metastasis, Hepatic Multiple				
Types	91	88	7.6	0.1
Pancreatic Cancer, (Head)	94	88	7.8	0.1
Renal Disease	24	88	2.0	0.9

	SENS	SPEC	LR +	LR -
PARATHYROID HORMONE				
C - TERMINAL ASSAY				
Primary Hyperparathyroidism	57-100*	95 - >99	11.4-100	<.1-0.5
N - TERMINAL ASSAY				
Primary Hyperparathyroidism	60-86*	95 - >99	12.0-86.0	0.1-0.4
INTACT				
Primary Hyperparathyroidism	55-100*	95 - >99	11.0-100	<.1-0.5

LR+ = Likelihood ratio of a Positive Test.
LR - = Likelihood ratio of a Negative Test.
* See reference notes for accurate interpretation.

	SENS	SPEC	LR +	LR -
PARTIAL THROMBOPLASTIN TIME (PTT)				
Hemophilia A				
Factor VIII Deficiency				
Severe*..................................	100	>99*	100	<.1
Moderate*...............................	99	>99*	99.0	<.1
Mild*......................................	90	>99*	90.0	0.1
von Willebrand Disease	48-100*	>99*	48.0-100	<.1-0.5
Hemophilia B				
Factor IX (Christmas)				
Deficiency.............................	100	>99*	100	<.1
Factor XII (Hageman)				
Deficiency	100*	>99*	100	<.1
Factor XI (Plasma Thrombo-				
plastin Antecedent)				
Deficiency.............................	100*	>99*	100	<.1
Factor X (Stuart-Prower)				
Deficiency.............................	100*	>99*	100	<.1

	SENS	SPEC	LR +	LR -
PM-1, NUCLEAR ANTIGENS				
CREST Syndrome.....................	<5	>95	1.0	1.0
Dermatomyositis	10	>95	2.0	0.9
Drug Induced Lupus	< 5	>95	1.0	1.0
Mixed Connective Tissue				
Disease....................................	< 5	>95	1.0	1.0
Polymyositis.............................	50-64	>95	10.0-12.8	0.4-0.5
Sjogren's Syndrome.................	<5	>95	1.0	1.0
Systemic Sclerosis...................	<5	>95	1.0	1.0
Systemic Lupus Erythematosus	<5	>95	1.0	1.0

	SENS	SPEC	LR +	LR -
PORPHOBILINOGEN				
MODIFIED WATSON-SCHWARTZ				
Porphyria				
(Acute Intermittent				
and Variegate)......................	100*	>99*	100	<.1
Liver Disease				
(Cirrhosis and Hepatitis).......	4	>99*	4.0	1.0
HOESCH				
Porphyria..................................	100*	>99*	100	<.1

LR+ = Likelihood ratio of a Positive Test.
LR - = Likelihood ratio of a Negative Test.
* See reference notes for accurate interpretation.

	SENS	SPEC	LR +	LR -
POTASSIUM				
Aldosteronism, Primary				
(all types).....................................	73	95	14.6	0.3
Adenoma*.....................................	80	95	16.0	0.2
Hyperplasia..................................	50	95	10.0	0.5

	SENS	SPEC	LR +	LR -
PROTHROMBIN TIME (PT)				
Factor VII Deficiency..................	100	>97	33.3	<.1

	SENS	SPEC	LR +	LR -
RANA (Rheumatoid Arthritis-Associated Nuclear Antigen)				
Rheumatoid Arthritis..................	85-95	>95	17.0-19	0.1-0.2

	SENS	SPEC	LR +	LR -
RENIN (SUPPRESSED)*				
Primary Aldosteronism...............	64*	83*	3.8	0.4

	SENS	SPEC	LR +	LR -
SCL 70				
CREST Syndrome......................	10-22	95	2.5-4.4	0.8-0.9
Dermatomyositis/Polymyositis..	< 5	95	1.0	1.0
Drug Induced Lupus	< 5	95	1.0	1.0
Mixed Connective Tissue				
Disease.....................................	< 5	95	1.0	1.0
Systemic Sclerosis....................	20-60	95	4.0-12.0	0.4-0.8
Systemic Lupus Erythematosus	< 5	95	1.0	1.0
Sjogren's Syndrome..................	< 5	95	1.0	1.0

	SENS	SPEC	LR +	LR -
SEROTONIN, URINARY EXCRETION				
Carcinoid*	64	98	32.0	0.4

	SENS	SPEC	LR +	LR -
SS-A ANTIBODY				
Dermatomyositis/Polymyositis..	10	95	2.0	0.9
Drug Induced Lupus	< 5	95	1.0	1.0
Mixed Connective Tissue				
Disease......................................	< 5	95	1.0	1.0

LR+ = Likelihood ratio of a Positive Test.
LR - = Likelihood ratio of a Negative Test.
* See reference notes for accurate interpretation.

(Cont.)	SENS	SPEC	LR +	LR -
Sjogren's Syndrome..................	< 5	95	1.0	1.0
Systemic Lupus				
Erythematosus..........................	25-40	95	5.0-8.0	0.6-0.8
Systemic Sclerosis....................	< 5	95	1.0	1.0

SS-B ANTIBODY				
CREST Syndrome......................	< 5	95	1.0	1.0
Dermatomyositis/Polymyositis..	< 5	95	1.0	1.0
Drug Induced Lupus	< 5	95	1.0	1.0
Mixed Connective Tissue				
Disease....................................	< 5	95	1.0	1.0
Sjogren's Syndrome..................	45-60	95	9.0-12.0	0.4-0.6
Systemic Lupus Erythematosus	5-15	95	1.0-3.0	0.9-1.0
Systemic Sclerosis....................	< 5	95	1.0	1.0

SS-DNA				
Systemic Lupus Erythematosus	60-70	> 95	12.0-14.0	0.3-0.4

THYROID ANTIMICROSOMAL ANTIBODIES				
Hemagglutination				
Graves' Disease........................	80-86	97	26.7-28.7	0.1-0.2
Hashimoto's Thyroiditis	95	97	31.7	0.1
Nontoxic Nodular Goiter..........	40*	97	13.3	0.6
Primary Hypothyroidism	84*	97	28.0	0.2

THYROID: ANTITHYRO-GLOBULIN ANTIBODIES-RIA*				
Graves' Disease (Treated)........	47	97	15.7	0.5
Graves' Disease (Untreated)....	55	97	18.3	0.5
Hashimoto's Thyroiditis	89*	97	29.7	0.1
Myxedema, Idiopathic	69*	97	23.0	0.3
Nontoxic Goiter..........................	10	97	3.3	0.9
Pituitary Hypothyroidism............	11*	97	3.7	0.9
Thyroid Cancer..........................	27	97	9.0	0.8
Toxic Adenoma	38	97	12.7	0.6

LR+ = Likelihood ratio of a Positive Test.
LR - = Likelihood ratio of a Negative Test.
* See reference notes for accurate interpretation.

	SENS	SPEC	LR +	LR -
THYROID: ANTITHYRO-GLOBULIN ANTIBODIES				
Hemagglutination*				
Graves' Disease (Treated)......	31	96	7.7	0.7
Graves' Disease (Untreated)..	22	96	5.4	0.8
Hashimoto's Thyroiditis..........	59-83*	96	14.8-20.8	0.2-0.4
Myxedema, Idiopathic..............	69*	96	17.3	0.3
Non-Toxic Goiter......................	7*	96	1.8	1.0
Pituitary Hypothyroidism.........	22	96	5.6	0.8
Thyroid Cancer........................	2	96	0.6	1.0
Toxic Adenoma	6	96	1.6	1.0
THYROID STIMULATING HORMONE				
TSH-RIA				
Hypothyroidism (Primary)........	100	92 - >99*	12.5 -100	<0.1
TSH-IRMA				
Hyperthyroidism......................	96	64 - >99*	2.7-96	<0.1
Hypothyroidism (Primary)........	100	>99	100	<0.1
TOTAL T4				
Hyperthyroidism......................	82-93	96 - >99*	20.5-93	0.1-.2
Hypothyroidism	44-93	81-98	2.3-46.5	0.1-0.7
FREE T4				
Hyperthyroidism......................	98-100	96-98	25-50	<0.1
Hypothyroidism	65	96-98	16.3-32.5	.4
FREE T4 INDEX				
Hyperthyroidism......................	61-88	96 - >99*	15.3-88	0.1-.4
Hypothyroidism	65	96-98	16.3-32.5	.4
TOTAL T3				
Hyperthyroidism......................	77 - 87	97-99*	25.7-87	0.1-.2
Hypothyroidism	23	98	11.5	0.8

LR+ = Likelihood ratio of a Positive Test.
LR - = Likelihood ratio of a Negative Test.
* See reference notes for accurate interpretation.

	SENS	SPEC	LR +	LR -
FREE T3				
Hyperthyroidism...............	94	98	47	0.1
Hypothyroidism	35	98	17.5	0.7

	SENS	SPEC	LR +	LR -
FREE T3 INDEX				
Hyperthyroidism...............	82-87	96 - >99	20.5-87	0.1-0.2
Hypothyroidism	29	95	5.8	0.7

	SENS	SPEC	LR +	LR -
TOTAL IRON BINDING CAPACITY (TIBC)				
Iron Deficiency Anemia *...........	71-82	61-92	1.8-10.3	0.2-0.5

	SENS	SPEC	LR +	LR -
TOXICOLOGY, URINE				
Amphetamines	19-100	63 - >99	0.5-100	<.1-1.3
Barbiturates..........................	11-94	94 - >99	1.8-94.0	0.1-0.9
Cocaine	0-100	94 - >99	0.0-100	<.1-1.1
Codeine	0-100	93 - >99	0.0-100	<.1-1.1
Methadone	0-33	34 - >99	0.0-33.0	0.7-2.9
Morphine	5-100	90 - >99	0.5-100	<.1-1.1

	SENS	SPEC	LR +	LR -
TRANSFERRIN*				
Hemochromatosis (<35 yrs.).....	82*	88*	6.8	0.2
Iron Deficiency Anemia *...........	66-83	61-79	1.7-4.0	0.2-0.6

	SENS	SPEC	LR +	LR -
TRYPSINOGEN				
Acute Pancreatitis	97	82* - >95	5.4-19.4	<.1

	SENS	SPEC	LR +	LR -
VANILLYLMANDELIC ACID (VMA), URINE				
Neuroblastoma............................	73*	>99*	73	0.3
Pheochromacytoma..................	89-95*	>99*	89.0-95.0	<.1

LR+ = Likelihood ratio of a Positive Test.
LR - = Likelihood ratio of a Negative Test.
* See reference notes for accurate interpretation.

	SENS	SPEC	LR +	LR -
VASOACTIVE INTESTINAL PEPTIDE				
VIPoma				
(Ganglioneuroblastoma)	100*	>99	100	<.1
VIPoma (Pancreas in adult)	100	>99	100	<.1

	SENS	SPEC	LR +	LR -
VDRL				
Primary Syphilis	76	84* - >99	4.8-76.0	0.2-0.3
Secondary Syphilis	74-100	84* - >99	4.6-100	<.1-0.3
Early-Latent (<1-2 yrs.) Syphilis	92*	84* - >99	5.8-92	0.1
Late-Latent (>2 yrs) Syphilis	77	84* - >99	4.8-77.0	0.2-0.3

WESTERN BLOT - (See Human Immunodeficiency Virus Tests)

LR+ = Likelihood ratio of a Positive Test.
LR - = Likelihood ratio of a Negative Test.
* See reference notes for accurate interpretation.

ACID PHOSPHATASE
1. Carson J.L., Eisenberg J.M., Shaw L.M., et al.: Diagnostic accuracy of four assays of prostatic acid phosphatase. *J.A.M.A.* 1985; 253(5):665-669.
2. Howard P.J., Fraley E.E.: Evaluation of the acid phosphatase in benign prostatic diseases. *J. Urology*, 1965; 94:687-90.
3. Vihko P., Kontturi M., Lukkarined O., et al.: Screening for carcinoma of the prostate. *Cancer* 1985; 56:173-77.
4. Gittes R.F.: Editorial retrospective: Serum acid phosphatase and screening for carcinoma of the prostate. *N. E. J. M.* 1983; 309(14): 852-53.

ALANINE AMINO TRANSFERASE
  (ALT, SGPT)
1. Ellis G., Goldberg D.M., Spooner R.J., et al.: Serum enzyme tests in diseases of the liver and biliary tree. *Am. J. Clin. Pathol.* 1978; 70(2):248-258.
2. Ferraris R., Colombatti C., Fiorentini M.T., et al.: Diagnostic value of serum bile acids and routine liver function tests in hepatobiliary diseases: Sensitivity, specificity and predictive value. *Digest. Dis. and Sci.* 1983; 28(2):129-136.
3. Liewendahl K., Schauman K.O.: Statistical evaluation of liver scanning in combination with liver function tests. *Acta Med. Scand.* 1972; 192:395-400.
4. Ferrante W.A., Maxfield W.S.: Comparison of the diagnostic accuracy of liver scans, liver function tests and liver biopsies. *Southern Med. J.* 1968; 61:1255-1263.

* N = 20 for carcinoma of the bile duct and N = 24 for primary biliary cirrhosis.
* specificity may be as low as 87 when testing populations with other disease processes. 95 = the specificity in "health."

ALDOSTERONE NONSUPPRESSED (concentration)
1. Bravo E.L., Tarazi R.C., Dustan H.P., et al.: The changing clinical spectrum of primary aldosteronism. *Am. J. Med.* 1983; 74:641-651.

* Nonsuppressed = elevated aldosterone despite 3 days of salt loading.
* Sensitivity and specificity are in relation to patients with essential
  hypertension and not to the general population (sensitivity would be
  higher when testing the normal population).
* N = 80, 70 patients with adrenal adenoma and 10 patients with adrenal
  hyperplasia.

ALDOSTERONE NONSUPPRESSED (excretion rate μg/24hrs)
1. Bravo E.L., Tarazi R.C., Dustan H.P., et al.: The changing clinical
   spectrum of primary aldosteronism. *Am. J. Med.* 1983; 74:641-651.

* Nonsuppressed = elevated aldosterone despite 3 days of salt loading.
* Sensitivity and specificity are in relation to patients with essential
  hypertension and not to the general population (sensitivity would be
  higher when testing the normal population).
* N = 80, 70 patients with adrenal adenoma and 10 patients with adrenal
  hyperplasia.

ALKALINE PHOSPHATASE
1. Ellis G., Goldberg D.M., Spooner R.J., et al.: Serum enzyme tests in
   diseases of the liver and biliary tree. *Am. J. Clin. Pathol.* 1978;
   70(2):248-258.
2. Jonsson P., Bengtsson G., Carlsson G., et al.: Value of serum-5-
   nucleotidase, alkaline phosphatase and gamma-glutamyl transferase
   for prediction of hepatic metastases preoperatively in colorectal
   cancer. *Acta. Chir. Scand.* 1984; 150:419-423.
3. Kowlessar O.D., Haeffner L.J., Riley E.M., et al.: Comparative study
   of serum leucine aminopeptidase, 5-nucleotidase and non-specific
   alkaline phosphatase in diseases affecting the pancreas, hepatobiliary tree and bone. *Am. J. Med.* 1961; 31:231-237.
4. Ferrante W.A., Maxfield W.S.: Comparison of the diagnostic accuracy
   of liver scans, liver function tests and liver biopsies. *Southern Med.
   J.* 1968; 61:1255-1263.

* N = 20 for Cancer of the bile duct, N = 27 for intrahepatic cholestasis
  and N = 24 for primary biliary cirrhosis.
* In colorectal cancer N = 25 for sensitivity. Specificity group was not
  from the "normal population" but patients with a previous diagnosis
  of colorectal cancer. Alkaline phosphatase demonstrated low
  sensitivity when < 1/4 of the liver volume was engaged by tumor and
  highly sensitive when > 3/4 of the liver volume was engaged by
  tumor. Population studied was Swedish.

ALPHA-FETOPROTEIN by Double Antibody RIA

1. Klavins J.V.: Advances in biological markers for cancer. *Annals Clin. Lab. Sci.* 1983; 13(4):275-280.
2. Waldmann T.A., McIntire K.R.: The use of a radioimmunoassay for alpha-fetoprotein in the diagnosis of malignancy. *Cancer.* 1974; 34:1510-1515.
3. Bloomer J.R., Waldmann T.A., McIntire K.R., et al.: Serum alpha-fetoprotein (AFP) in non-neoplastic liver diseases. *Clinical Research.* 1974; 22:354A.
4. Kurman R.J., Scardino P.T., McIntire K.R., et al.: Cellular localization of alpha-fetoprotein and human chorionic gonadotropin in germ cell tumors of the testis using an indirect immunoperoxidase technique. *Cancer.* 1977; 40:2136-2151.

AMMONIA

1. Fazekas J.F., Ticktin H.E., Ehrmantraut W.R., et al.: Cerebral metabolism in hepatic insufficiency. *Am. J. Med.* 1956; 21:843-849.
2. Glasgow A.M., Cotton R.B., Dhiensiri K., et al.: Reye's syndrome. *Amer. J. Dis. Child.* 1972; 124:827-833.
3. Bakerman S.: *A B C's of Laboratory Data* (2nd ed.). Interpretive laboratory data 1984; p33.

* Reference #1 states that arterial and venous blood ammonia values were not significantly different (n = 7 for those tested at both sites). Reference #1 used arterial samples for their data. Reference #2 used venous blood. Reference #3 suggests venous blood.
* Cut off values vary with age. * N = 12 for "hepatic insufficiency without cerebral dysfunction", N = 8 for "with cerebral dysfunction", N = 11 for hepatic coma.

AMYLASE

1. Steinberg W.M., Goldstein S.S., Davis N.D., et al.:Diagnostic assays in acute pancreatitis. *Annals Int. Med.* 1985; 102:576-580.
2. Eckfeldt J.H., Kolars J.C., Elson M.K., et al.: Serum tests for pancreatitis in patients with abdominal pain. *Arch. Pathol. Lab. Med.* 1985; 109:316-319.
3. Stefanini P., Ermini M., Carboni M.: Diagnosis and management of acute pancreatitis. *Am. J. Surg.* 1965; 110:866-875.

* The specificity of 89 is from a control group of patients with abdominal pain. Specificity may be as low as 71 when control group is composed of those with suspected pancreatitis or from a population with a high frequency of chronic medical disease.

ANTI-NUCLEAR ANTIBODY
1. Harmon C.E.: Antinuclear antibodies in autoimmune disease. *Medical Clinics of N. Am.* 1985; 69(3):547-563.
2. Tan E.M., Robinson C.A., Nakamura R.M.: ANAs in systemic rheumatic disease. *Postgrad. Med.* 1985; 76(3):141-148.
3. Calabrese L.H.: Diagnosis of systemic lupus erythematosus. *Postgrad. Med.* 1984; 75(7):103-112.

* Specificity is 69 when testing in patients clinically suspected of having rheumatic disease and 95 when testing in the "healthy" population. The predictive value of a positive test is much higher in the former.

ANTI-RIBONUCLEAR PROTEIN
1. Sharp G.C., Irvin W.S., May C.M., et al.: Association of antibodies to ribonucleoprotein and Sm antigens with mixed connective-tissue disease, systemic lupus erythematosus and other rheumatic diseases, *N.E.J.M.* 1976; 295(21):1149-1154.
2. Harmon C.E.: Antinuclear antibodies in autoimmune disease. *Medical Clinics of N. Am.* 1985; 69(3):547-563.
3. Tan E.M., Robinson C.A., Nakamura R.M.: ANAs in systemic rheumatic disease. *Postgrad. Med.* 1985; 76(3):141-148.
4. Notman D.D., Kurata N., Tan E.M.: Profiles of antinuclear antibodies in systemic rheumatic diseases. *Ann Int. Med.* 1975; 83:464-469.
5. Tan E.M.: Antinuclear antibodies in diagnosis and management. *Hosp. Pract.* 1983:79-84.

ANTI-SM ANTIBODY
1. Notman D.D., Kurata N., Tan E.M.: Profiles of antinuclear antibodies in systemic rheumatic diseases. *Ann Int. Med.* 1975; 83:464-469.
2. Harmon C.E.: Antinuclear antibodies in autoimmune disease. *Medical Clinics of N. Am.* 1985; 69(3):547-563.
3. Tan E.M., Robinson C.A., Nakamura R.M.: ANAs in systemic rheumatic disease. *Postgrad. Med.* 1985; 76(3):141-148.
4. Tan E.M.: Antinuclear antibodies in diagnosis and management. *Hosp. Pract.* Jan.1983:79-84.

ANTITHROMBIN III

1. Weimer, C.P., Brandt, J.: Plasma antithrombin III activity: An aid in the diagnosis of preeclampsia-eclampsia. *Am. J. Ob. Gyn.* 1982; 142(3): 275-281.
2. Weimer, C.P., Kwaan, H.C., Paul, M., et al: Antithrombin III activity in women with hypertension during pregnancy, *Ob. Gyn.* 1985; 65(3): 301-306.
3. Spero, J.A., Lewis, J.H., Hasiba, U.: Disseminated Intravascular Coagulation: findings in 346 Patients. *Thromb. Haemost* 1980; 43(1):28-33.

* Control Group for specificity includes females at 35-37 weeks gestation.
* Patients were post surgery from a variety of procedures including coronary bypass and aortic aneurysm repair.
* Liver disease group includes 36% with acute liver failure, 36% with chronic liver disease and 28% with unknown cause. N= 27 for liver disease group.

ASPARTATE AMINOTRANSFERASE
(AST, SGOT)

1. Ellis G., Goldberg D.M., Spooner R.J., et al.: Serum enzyme tests in diseases of the liver and biliary tree. *Am. J. Clin. Pathol.* 1978; 70(2):248-258.
2. Ferraris R., Colombatti C., Fiorentini M.T., et al.: Diagnostic value of serum bile acids and routine liver function tests in hepatobiliary diseases: Sensitivity, specificity and predictive value. *Digest. Dis. and Sci.* 1983; 28(2):129-136.
3. Lee T.H., Cook E.F., Weisberg M., et al.: Acute chest pain in the emergency room. *Arch. Int. Med.* 1985; 145:65-69.
4. Liewendahl K., Schauman K.O.: Statistical evaluation of liver scanning in combination with liver function tests. *Acta Med. Scand.* 1972; 192:395-400.
5. Ferrante W.A., Maxfield W.S.: Comparison of the diagnostic accuracy of liver scans, liver function tests and liver biopsies. *Southern Med. J.* 1968; 61:1255-1263.
6. Mayer A.D., McMahon M.J.: Biochemical identification of patients with gallstones associated with acute pancreatitis on the day of admission to hospital. *Ann. Surg.* 1984; 201(1):68-75.
7. Lee, T.H., Goldman, L.: Serum enzyme assays in the diagnosis of acute myocardial infarction, *Annals of Int. Med.* 1986;105:221-33.

8. Lee, T.H., Weisberg, M.C., Cook, E.F., et al: Evaluation of creatine kinase and creatine kinase-MB for diagnosing myocardial infarction, *Arch Intern Med,* 1987; 147: 115-121.

* N = 20 for carcinoma of the bile duct and N = 24 for primary biliary cirrhosis.
* Specificity may be as low as 87 when testing populations with other disease processes. 99 = the specificity in "health".
* Sensitivity has been shown to be higher when levels are obtained 12 hours after onset of symptoms, and lower when less than 12 hours. Population used for specificity (N= 82) was composed of patients presenting to the emergency room with chest pain.

ASPARTATE AMINOTRANSFERASE, Serial Tests
1. Lee, T.H., Goldman, L.: Serum enzyme assays in the diagnosis of acute myocardial infarction, *Annals of Int. Med.* 1986; 105:221-33.
2. Grande, P., Christiansen, C., Pedersen, A.: Optimal diagnosis in acute myocardial infarction, *Circulation,* 1980; 61(4) 723-728.

* Serial tests defined as three samples obtained at 12 hour intervals.

B$_{12}$
1. Griner F.P., Oranburg P. R.: Predictive values of erythrocyte indices for tests of iron, folic acid and vitamin B$_{12}$ deficiency. *A.J.C.P.* 1978; 70(5):748-752.

* When MCV > 95 the probability of either a low B$_{12}$ or folate is 0.18.

BILE ACIDS (Fasting)
1. Ferraris R., Colombatti C., Fiorentini M.T., et al.: Diagnostic value of serum bile acids and routine liver function tests in hepatobiliary diseases: Sensitivity, specificity and predictive value. *Digest. Dis. and Sci.* 1983; 28(2):129-136.
2. Cravetto,C., Molino,G., Biondi,A.M.: Evaluation of the diagnostic value of serum bile acid in the detection and functional assessment of liver diseases *Ann. Clin. Biochem.* 1985; 22:596-605.

* Specificity may be as low as 88 when testing populations with other disease processes. 99 = the specificity in "health."

BILIRUBIN, TOTAL

1. Ferraris R., Colombatti C., Fiorentini M.T., et al.: Diagnostic value of serum bile acids and routine liver function tests in hepatobiliary diseases: Sensitivity, specificity and predictive value. *Digest. Dis. and Sci.* 1983; 28(2):129-136.
2. Gollin F.F., Sims J.L., Cameron J.R.: Liver scanning and liver function tests. *J.A.M.A..* 1964; 187(2):111-116.

BLEEDING TIME

1. Lian, E.C., Deykin, D.: Diagnosis of von Willebrand's disease, A comparative study of diagnostic tests on nine families with von Willebrand's disease and its differential diagnosis from hemophilia and thrombocytopathy. *Am. J. of Med.* 1976; 60:344-356.
2. Bain, B., Forster, T., Baker, A.: An assessment of the sensitivity of 3 bleeding time techniques. *Scand. J. Haematol.* 1983; 30:311-316.
3. Lind, S.E.: Prolonged Bleeding Time. *Am. J. of Med.* 1984; 77:305-309.

C-PEPTIDE

1. Koskinen, P., Viikari, J., Irjala, K., et. al.: Plasma and urinary C-peptide in the classification of adult diabetics. *Scand. J. Clin. Lab. Invest.* 1986; 46:655-663.

* Specificity was obtained from type II diabetics.

C-PEPTIDE Glucagon Stimulation Test

1. Koskinen, P., Viikari, J., Irjala, K., et. al.: Plasma and urinary C-peptide in the classification of adult diabetics. *Scand. J. Clin. Lab. Invest.* 1986; 46:655-663.

* Specificity was obtained from type II diabetics.

C-REACTIVE PROTEIN

1. Mallya, A.K., deBeer, F.C., Berry, H., et al.: Correlation of clinical parameters of disease activity in rheumatoid arthritis with serum concentration of C-Reactive protein and erythrocyte sedimentation rate. *J. of Rheum.,* 1982; 9(2):224-228.
2. Kaplan E.L., Wannamaker, L.W.,: C-Reactive protein in streptococcal pharyngitis. *Pediatrics,* 1977; 60(1):28-32.

3. Peltola, H.: C-Reactive protein in rapid differentiation of acute epiglottitis from spasmodic croup and acute laryngotracheitis: A preliminary report. *J. Pediatrics.* 1983; 102(50):713-715.
4. deBeer, F.C., Kirsten, G.F., Gie, R.P., et al: Value of C-Reactive protein measurement in tuberculosis, bacterial, and viral meningitis. *Arch. of Dis. in Child.* 1984; 59:653-656.
5. Clark, D., Cost, K.: Use of Serum C-Reactive protein in differentiating septic from aseptic meningitis in children. *J. of Pediatrics.* 1983; 102(5):718-720.

* N= 5 for mild (grade 1) rheumatoid arthritis, N = 10 for severe (grade 4) rheumatoid arthritis.
* Severity score is based on subjective *ie.* amount of pain and stiffness and semiobjective *ie.* ESR, hemoglobin, articular index, etc. information.
* Specificity = 47 in patients with pharyngitis which is not streptococcal. Specificity = 99 in the healthy population.
* Specificity = 88 in patients with laryngotracheitis or spasmodic croup. N = 10 for sensitivity.
* Some studies advocate the use of C-Reactive Protein in differentiating bacterial from viral meningitis. Levels may also be elevated in meningitis due to tuberculosis.

CALCIUM

1. Valsamis, J., Van Peborgh, J., Brauman, H.: Relative contribution of various expressions of cAMP excretion to other indices of parathyroid function, as tested by discriminant multivariate linear regression analysis. *Clin. Chem.* 1986; 32(7):1279-1284.
2. Arnaud, C.D., Goldsmith, R.S., Bordier, P.J., et. al.: Influence of Immunoheterogeneity of circulating parathyroid hormone on results of radioimmunoassays of serum in man. *Am. J. of Med.* 1974; 56:785-793.
3. Hawker, C.D.: Parathyroid hormone: radioimmunoassay and clinical interpretation. *Ann. of Clin. and Lab. Sci.* 1975; 5(5):383-398.

cAMP

1. Broadus, A.E., Mahaffey, J.E., Barter, F.C., et al,: Nephrogenous cyclic adenosine monophosphate as a parathyroid function test, *J. Clin. Invest.* 1977; 60:771-83.
2. Dohan, P.H., Yamashita, K., Larsen, P.E., et al: Evaluation of urinary cyclic 3' 5'-adenosine monophosphate excretion in the differential diagnosis of hypercalcemia. *J. Clin. Endo. and Metab.* 1972; 35:775-784.
3. Valsamis, J., Van Peborgh, J., Brauman, H.: Relative contribution of various expressions of cAMP excretion to other indices of parathyroid function, as tested by discriminant multivariate linear regression analysis. *Clin. Chem.* 1986; 32(7):1279-1284.

CARCINOEMBYRONIC ANTIGEN

1. Gail M.H., Muenz L., Mcintire K.R., et al.: Multiple markers for lung cancer diagnsis: Validation of models for advanced cancer. *JNCI.* 1986; 76(5):805-816.
2. Galen, R.S., Gambino, S.R. Beyond Normality: The Predictive Value and Efficiency of Medical Diagnoses. New York, John Wiley and Sons, 1975.

CAROTENE

1. Luk, G.D.: Computer assisted multivariate analysis of serum carotene, albumin, cholesterol, and prothrombin time as screening tests for fat malabsorption. *Gastroenterology,* 1979; 76:1189.
2. Naveh, Y., Ken-Dror, A., Zinder, O.: Comparative reliability of D-xylose absorption and serum beta-carotene measurements in small intestinal disease. *J. Ped. Gastroenterol. Nutr.* 1986; 5(2): 210-3.

CATECHOLAMINES

1. Sjoerdsma, A., Engelman, K., Waldmann,T.A.: Pheochromocytoma: Current concepts of diagnosis and treatment. *Ann. Int. Med.,* 1966; 65(6):1302-1325.
2. Kaufman, B.H., Telander, R.L., van Heerden, J.A.: Pheochromocytoma in the pediatric age group: current status, *J. of Ped. Surg.* 1983; 18(6);879-883.
3. van Heerden J.A., Sheps S.G., Hamberger B., et. al.: Pheochromocytoma: Current status and changing trends. *Surgery,* 1982; 91(4):367-73.

4. Bravo E.L., Tarazi R.C., Gifford R.W., et al.: Circulating and urinary catecholamines in pheochromocytoma: Diagnostic and pathophysiologic implications. *N. J. E. M.* 1979; 301(13):682-686.
5. Bravo, E.L., Gifford, R.W.: Pheochromacytoma: Diagnosis, localization and management. *N.E.J.M.* 1984;311(20):1298-1302.

* Specificity=95 calculated from patients with essential hypertension.

CENTROMERE/KINETOCHORE

1. Harmon, C.E.: Antinuclear antibodies in autoimmune disease, significance and pathogenicity, *Symposium on Clinical Immunology I,* 1985; 69(3):547-563.
2. Tan, E.M., Robinson, C.A., Nakamura, R.M.: ANAs in systemic rheumatic disease. *Postgrad. Med.* 1985; 78(3):141-148.
3. Tan, E.M.: Antinuclear antibodies in diagnosis and management. *Hosp Pract.* 1983; 79-84.

CERULOPLASMIN

1. Sass-Kortsak, A.: Wilson's disease a treatable liver disease in children. *Ped Clinics of No. Am.* 1975; 22(4):963-984.
2. Sternlieb, I., Scheinberg, I.H.: Prevention of Wilson's disease in asymptomatic patients. *N.E.J.M.* 1968; 278:352-359.
3. LaRusso, N.F., Summerskill, W.H.J., McCall, J.T.: Abnormalities of chemical tests for copper metabolism in chronic active liver disease: differentiation from Wilson's disease. *Gastroenterology* 1976; 70(5):653-655.
4. Sternlieb, I.: Diagnosis of Wilson's Disease. *Gastroenterology* 1978; 74(4):787-789.
5. Summer, K.H., Eisenburg, J.: Low content of hepatic reduced glutathione in patients with Wilson's disease. *Biochem. Med.* 1985; 34:107-111.

COPPER

1. Sass-Kortsak, A.: Wilson's disease a treatable liver disease in children. *Ped Clinics of No. Am.* 1975; 22(4):963-984.
2. Sternlieb, I., Scheinberg, I.H.: Prevention of Wilson's disease in asymptomatic patients. *N.E.J.M.* 1968; 278:352-359.
3. LaRusso, N.F., Summerskill, W.H.J., McCall, J.T.: Abnormalities of chemical tests for copper metabolism in chronic active liver disease: differentiation from Wilson's disease. *Gastroenterology* 1976; 70(5):653-655.

4. Sternlieb, I.: Diagnosis of Wilson's Disease. *Gastroenterology* 1978; 74(4):787-789.

Copper, µg/24 hr. urine
1. Sass-Kortsak, A.: Wilson's disease a treatable liver disease in children. *Ped Clinics of No. Am.* 1975; 22(4):963-984.
2. Sternlieb, I., Scheinberg, I.H.: Prevention of Wilson's disease in asymptomatic patients. *N.E.J.M.* 1968; 278:352-359.
3. LaRusso, N.F., Summerskill, W.H.J., McCall, J.T.: Abnormalities of chemical tests for copper metabolism in chronic active liver disease: differentiation from Wilson's disease. *Gastroenterology* 1976; 70(5): 653-655.
4. Sternlieb, I.: Diagnosis of Wilson's Disease. *Gastroenterology* 1978; 74(4):787-789.
5. Summer, K.H., Eisenburg, J.: Low content of hepatic reduced glutathione in patients with Wilson's disease. *Biochem. Med.* 1985; 34:107-111.

CORTISOL, 24 hour FREE URINE
1. Crapo L: Cushing's Syndrome: A review of diagnostic tests. *Metab.* 1979; 28:955-977.
2. Dunlap NE, Grizzle WE, Seigel AL: Cushing's Syndrome: Screening methods in hospitalized patients. *Arch. Path. Lab. Med.* 1985; 109:222-229.

CORTISOL, PLASMA
1. Crapo L: Cushing's Syndrome: A review of diagnostic tests. *Metab.* 1979; 28:955-977.
2. Eddy RL: Cushing's Syndrome: A prospective study of diagnostic methods. *Am. J. Med.* 1973; 55:621-630.
3. Ernest I: Steroid excretion and plasma cortisol in 41 cases of Cushing's Syndrome. *Acta. Endocrin.* 1966; 51:511-525.
4. Dunlap NE, Grizzle WE, Seigel AL: Cushing's Syndrome: Screening methods in hospitalized patients. *Arch. Path. Lab. Med.* 1985; 109:222-229.

CREATININE PHOSPHOKINASE MB Fraction, Single Test
1. Lee, T.H., Goldman, L.: Serum enzyme assays in the diagnosis of acute myocardial infarction, *Annals of Int. Med,* 1986; 105:221-33.
2. Lee, T.H., Weisberg, M.C., Cook, E.F., et al: Evaluation of creatine kinase and creatine kinase-MB for diagnosing myocardial infarction, *Arch Intern Med,* 1987; 147:115-121.

CREATINE PHOSPHOKINASE, MB FRACTION Serial Tests
1. Lee, T.H., Goldman, L.: Serum enzyme assays in the diagnosis of acute myocardial infarction, *Annals of Int. Med.* 1986; 105:221-33.
2. Grande, P., Christiansen, C., Pedersen, A.: Optimal diagnosis in acute myocardial infarction, *Circulation,* 1980; 61(4) 723-728.

* Serial tests are defined as three samples obtained at 12 hour intervals.
* Black and Hispanic individuals may show elevated normal values.

CREATINE PHOSPHOKINASE, TOTAL, Single Tests
1. Lee, T.H., Goldman, L.: Serum enzyme assays in the diagnosis of acute myocardial infarction, *Annals of Int. Med.* 1986; 105:221-33.
2. Lee, T.H., Weisberg, M.C., Cook, E.F., et al: Evaluation of creatine kinase and creatine kinase-MB for diagnosing myocardial infarction, *Arch. Intern. Med.* 1987; 147:115-121.
3. Grande, P., Christiansen, C., Pedersen, A.: Optimal diagnosis in acute myocardial infarction, *Circulation,* 1980; 61(4) 723-728.

* Black and Hispanic individuals may show elevated normal values.

CREATINE PHOSPHOKINASE, TOTAL, Serial Tests
1. Lee, T.H., Goldman, L.: Serum enzyme assays in the diagnosis of acute myocardial infarction, *Annals of Int. Med.* 1986; 105:221-33.
2. Grande, P., Christiansen, C., Pedersen, A.: Optimal diagnosis in acute myocardial infarction, *Circulation,* 1980; 61(4)723-728.

* Serial tests are defined as three samples obtained at 12 hour intervals.
* Black and Hispanic individuals may show elevated normal values.

DEXAMETHASONE HIGH DOSE (2mg) SUPPRESSION - TWO DAY and DEXAMETHASONE SUPPRESSION - OVERNIGHT
1. Crapo L: Cushing's Syndrome: A review of diagnostic tests. *Metab.* 1979; 28:955-977.
2. Dunlap NE, Grizzle WE, Seigel AL: Cushing's Syndrome: Screening methods in hospitalized patients. *Arch. Path. Lab. Med.* 1985; 109:222-229.

3. Liddle GW: Tests of adrenal-pituitary suppressibility in the diagnosis of Cushing's Syndrome. *J Clin Endo. and Metab.* 1960; 20:1539-1560.
4. Tyrrell, J.B., Findling, J.W., Aron, D.C., et al: An overnight high-dose dexamethasone suppression test for rapid differential diagnosis of Cushing's Syndrome. *Ann. Int. Med.* 1986; 104:180-186.

DNA, Double Stranded

1. Harmon, C.E.: Antinuclear antibodies in autoimmune disease, significance and pathogenicity, *Symposium on Clinical Immunology I*, 1985; 69(3):547-563.
2. Tan, E.M., Robinson, C.A., Nakamura, R.M.: ANAs in systemic rheumatic disease. *Postgrad. Med.* 1985; 78(3):141-148.
3. Tan, E.M., from *Advances in Immunology,* Kunkle and Dixon (eds.), Vol. 33, 1982; 172-185.
4. Nakamura, R.M., Rippey, J.H.: Quality assurance and proficiency testing for autoantibodies to nuclear antigen. *Arch. Pathol. Lab. Med.* 1985; 109:109-114.
5. Tan, E.M.: Antinuclear antibodies in diagnosis and management. *Hosp Pract.* 1983; 79-84.
6. Koffler, D., Miller, T.E., Faiferman, I.: Antipolynucleotide antibodies, the rheumatic connection. *Human Path.* 1983; 14(5):406-418.

DNA, Single Stranded

1. Harmon, C.E.: Antinuclear antibodies in autoimmune disease, significance and pathogenicity, *Symposium on Clinical Immunology I,* 1985; 69(3):547-563.
2. Tan, E.M., from *Advances in Immunology,* Kunkle and Dixon (eds.), Vol. 33, 1982; 172-185.
3. Nakamura, R.M., Rippey, J.H.: Quality assurance and proficiency testing for autoantibodies to nuclear antigen. *Arch. Pathol. Lab. Med.* 1985; 109:109-114.
4. Koffler, D., Miller, T.E., Faiferman, I.: Antipolynucleotide antibodies, the rheumatic connection. *Human Path.* 1983; 14(5):406-418.

ERYTHROCYTE PROTOPORPHYRIN (Epp)

1. Hershko, C., Bar-Or, D., Gaziel, Y.: Diagnosis of iron deficiency anemia in a rural population of children. Relative usefulness of serum ferritin, red cell protoporphyrin, red cell indices, and transferrin saturation determinations. *Am. J. of Clin. Nut.* 1981; 34:1600-1610.

2. Walsh J.R., Fredreckson M.: Serum ferritin, free erythrocyte protoporphyrin, and urinary iron excretion in patients with iron disorders. *Am. J. Med. Sci.* 1977; 273(3):293-300.

* The sensitivity and specificity values were obtained from children ages 1-6 (ref. #1). There is further evidence of similar utility in adults (see ref. #2).

FECAL FAT and TRIOLEIN BREATH TEST
1. Luk, G.D.: Qualitative Fecal Fat by Light Microscopy: A Sensitive and Specific screening test for steatorrhea and pancreatic insufficiency. *Gastroenterology* 1979; 76:1189.
2. Newcomer, A.D.,Hofmann, A.F.,DiMagno,E.P.:Triolein Breath Test for fat malabsorption. *Gastroenterology.* 1979; 76(1):6-13.
3. Bin,T.L.,Stoppard,M., Anderson,S. Assessment of fat malabsorption. *J. Clin. Pathol.* 1983; 36:1362-1366.

FERRITIN
1. Bassett M.L., Halliday J.W., Ferris R.A., et al.: Diagnosis of hemochromatosis in young subjects: Predictive accuracy of biochemical screening tests, *Gastroenterology.* 1984; 87:628-633.
2. Borwein S.T., Ghent C.N., Valberg L.S.: Diagnostic efficacy of screening tests for hereditary hemochromatosis. *Can. Med. Assoc. J.* 1984; 131:895-901.
3. Hershko, C., Bar-Or, D., Gaziel, Y.: Diagnosis of iron deficiency anemia in a rural population of children. Relative usefulness of serum ferritin, red cell protoporphyrin, red cell indices, and transferrin saturation determinations. *Am J. of Clin. Nut.* 1981; 34:1600-1610.
4. Walsh J.R., Fredreckson M.: Serum ferritin, free erythrocyte protoporphyrin, and urinary iron excretion in patients with iron disorders. *Am. J. Med. Sci.* 1977; 273(3):293-300.
5. Mazza J., Barr R.M., McDonald J.W., et. al.: Usefulness of the serum ferritin concentration in the detection of iron deficiency in a general hospital. *CMA. J.* 1978; 119:884-886.
6. Kalmin N.D., Robson E.B., Bettigole R.E.: Serum ferritin and marrow iron stores. *N.Y. State J. Med.* 1978; June:1052-1055.

* The sensitivity and specificity values for iron deficiency anemia were obtained from children ages 1-6 (ref. #1). There is further evidence of similar utility in adults (see ref. #4-6). The specificity of ferritin is thought to be higher in adults vs. transferrin (96 vs. 63 respectively, see ref.#5).

FIBRINOGEN/FIBRIN FRAGMENT - RIA

1. Zielinsky A., Hirsh J., Straumanis G., et al.: The diagnostic value of the fibrinogen/fibrin fragment E antigen assay in clinically suspected deep vein thrombosis. *Blood* 1982; 59(2):346-350.

* Use in ambulatory patients is preferred. Inpatient testing has a high false positive rate, especially post surgical patients. Specificity in ambulatory patients = 84, inpatients = 65.

FOLIC ACID

1. Griner F.P., Oranburg P. R.: Predictive values of erythrocyte indices for tests of iron, folic acid and vitamin B_{12} deficiency. *A.J.C.P.* 1978; 70(5):748-752.

* When MCV > 95 the probability of either a low B_{12} or folate is 0.18.

FSH

1. Yen S.S., Tsai C.C., Vandenburg G., et al.: Gonadotropin dynamics in patients with gonadal dysgenesis: A model for the study of gonadotropin regulation. *J. Clin. Endo and Metab.* 1972; 35(6):897-904.
2. Deutsch S., Krumholz B., Benjamin I.: *J. Reprod. Med.* 1978; 20(5):275-282.

* Specificity is from menstruating premenopausal women during the first half of the follicular phase of the cycle.

FTA-AB

1. Moyer N.P., Hudson J.D., Hausler W.J.: Evaluation of the bio-enzabead test for syphilis. *J. Clin. Microbiol.* 1987; 25(4):619-923.
2. Moyer N.P., Hudson J.D., Hausler W.J.: Evaluation of the hemagglutination treponemal test for syphilis. *J. Clin. Microbiol.* 1984; 19(6):849-852.
3. Deacon W.E., Lucas J.B., Price E.V.: Fluorescent treponemal antibody-absorption (FTA-ASB) test for syphilis. *J.A.M.A.*, 1966; 198,No 6:624-628.
4. Hart, G.: Syphilis tests in diagnostic and therapeutic decision making. *Ann. of Int. Med.* 1986; 104:368-376.

* When testing previously treated subjects sensitivity does not decrease more than 7% in any group.
* Specificity may be as low as 77 when testing populations with other illnesses.

GAMMA-GLUTAMYLTRANSPEPTIDASE

1. Cravetto C., Molino G., Biondi A.M., et al.: Evaluation of the diagnostic value of serum bile acid in the detection and functional assessment of liver diseases. *Ann. Clin. Biochem.* 1985; 22:596-605.
2. Rutenburg A. M., Goldbarg J. A., Pineda E. P.,: Serum gamma-glutamyl transpeptidase activity in hepatobiliary pancreatic disease. *Gastroenterology* 1963; 45(1):43-48.
3. Aronsen K. F., Nosslin B., Pihl B.: The value of Gamma-glutamyl transferase as a screen test for liver tumor. *Acta Chir. Scand.* 1970; 136:17-22.

* The group labeled as "liver disease" included: alcoholic hepatitis, chronic persistent hepatitiis, chronic active hepatitis, compensated cirrhosis, ascitic cirrhosis, primary biliary cirrhosis, obstructive jaundice, and acute viral hepatitis.
* There is a general rise in sensitivity when the disease process has associated jaundice.

GROWTH HORMONE - 2 Hour Glucagon Stimulation Test

1. Mitchell M.L., Byrne M.J., Sanchez Y., *et al.*: Detection of growth-hormone deficiency: The glucagon stimulation test. *N.E.J.M.* 1970; 282(10):539-41.

* The test is positive when growth hormone does not increase to normal range 2 hours post glucagon administration.

GROWTH HORMONE - 1 Hour Post Oral Glucose Load

1. Earll J.M., Sparks L.L., Forsham P.H. : Glucose suppression of serum growth hormone in the diagnosis of acromegaly. *J.A.M.A.* 1967; 201:628-30.

* Note: sensitivity from N = 14,specificity from N= 8. The test is abnormal when growth hormone is above the normal range for 1 hour post glucose load.

HAPTOGLOBIN
1. Marchand A., Galen R.S., Van Lente F.: The predictive value of serum haptoglobin in hemolytic disease. *J.A.M.A.* 1980; 243(19): 1909-1911.
2. Nosslin B.F., Nyman M.: Haptoglobin determination in the diagnosis of haemolytic diseases. *Lancet* 1958; 1:1000-1001.

* Megaloblastic anemia and hypersplenism showed less sensitivity than other hemolytic disorders.
* The specificity is in relation to those with nonhemolytic anemia not to normal controls.

HEMOGLOBIN A1C
1. Schwartz J.S., Clancy C.M.: Glycosylated hemoglobin assays in the management and diagnosis of diabetes mellitus. *Ann. Int. Med.* 1984; 101:710-713.
2. Simon D., Coignet M.C., Thibult N., et al.: Comparison of glycosylated hemoglobin and fasting plasma glucose with two-hour post-load plasma glucose in the detection of diabetes mellitus. *Am. J. Epid.* 1985; 122(4):589-593.
3. Baxi L., Barad D., Reece E.A.: Use of glycosylated hemoglobin as a screen for macrosomia in gestational diabetes. *Ob. & Gyn.* 1984; 64(3):347-350.

* Population studied for sensitivity and specificity is from Paris, France.

HEPATITIS A ANTIBODY TESTS
1. Storch G.A., Bodicky C., Blecka L.J., et al.: Use of conventional and IgM-specific RIA for anti-hepatitis A antibody in an outbreak of hepatitis A. *Am. J. Med.* 1982; 73:663-668.
2. Polesky H.F., Hanson M.R.: Comparison of viral hepatitis marker test methods based on AABB-CAP survey data. *AM. Soc. Clin. Path.* 1981; 76:521-524.
3. Czaja A.J. Serologic markers of hepatitis A and B in acute and chronic liver disease. *Mayo Clin. Proc.* 1979; 54:721-732.

HEPATITIS B ANTIBODY AND ANTIGEN TESTS

1. Ratnam S., Tobin A.M.: Comparative evaluation of commercial enzyme immunoassay kits for detection of hepatitis B seromarkers. *J. Clin. Mircobiol.* 1987; 25:432-433.
2. Polesky H.F., Hanson M.R.: Comparison of viral hepatitis marker test methods based on AABB-CAP survey Data. *Am. Soc. Clin. Path.* 1981; 76:521-524.
3. Czaja A.J. Serologic markers of hepatitis A and B in acute and chronic liver disease. *Mayo Clin. Proc.* 1979; 54:721-732.
4. Holland P. Hepatitis B surface antigen and antibody. Hepatitis B. *Academic Press* 1985, pp 5-25.

HETEROPHILE ANTIBODY

1. Evans A.S., Niederman J. C., Cenbre L.C., et al.: A prospective evaluation of heterophile and Epstein-Barr virus-specific IgM antibody tests in clinical and subclinical infectious mononucleosis: Specificity and sensitivity of the tests and persistence of antibody. *J. Infect. Dis.* 1975; 132(5):546-554.
2. Hoiby E.A., Tjade T., Rotterud J.: Evaluation of ten commercial heterophile antibody tests for infectious mononucleosis. *Acta Path. Microbio. Immuno. Scand.* 1985; 93:145-51.

* Sensitivity is given as a range representing the first week of acute infection to the third week of infection.
* Reference #2 demonstrates significant variation in sensitivity and specificity among the various commercially available agglutination kits.

HISTONES

1. Harmon, C.E.: Antinuclear antibodies in autoimmune disease, significance and pathogenicity, *Symposium on Clinical Immunology I,* 1985; 69(3):547-563.
2. Tan, E.M., Robinson, C.A., Nakamura, R.M.: ANAs in systemic rheumatic disease. *Postgrad. Med.* 1985; 78(3):141-148.
3. Tan, E.M.,: *Advances in Immunology,* Kunkle and Dixon (eds.), Vol. 33, 1982; 172-185.
4. Tan, E.M.: Antinuclear antibodies in diagnosis and management. *Hosp Pract.* 1983; 79-84.

HLA-B27
1. Calin A.: HLA-B27 in 1982: Reappraisal of a clinical test . *Ann. Int. Med.* 1982; 96(1):114-115.
2. Khan M.A., Khan M.K.: Diagnostic value of HLA-B27 testing in ankylosing spondylitis and Reiter's syndrome. *Ann. Int. Med.* 1982; 96;70-76.
3. Hawkins B.R., Dawkins R.L., Christiansen F.T., et al.: Use of the B27 test in the diagnosis of ankylosing spondylitis: A statistical evaluation. *Arthritis and Rheumat.* 1981; 24(5):743-746.

HOMOVANILIC ACID (24 HOUR URINE)
1. Tuchman M., Ramnaranine M.L., Woods W.G., et al.: Three years of experience with random urinary homovanilic and vanillylmandelic acid levels in the diagnosis of neuroblastoma. *Peds.* 1987; 79(2):203-205.
2. Kaufman B.H., Telander R.L., van Heerden J.A., et al.: Pheochromocytoma in the pediatric age group: Current status. *J. Ped. Surg.* 1983; 18(6):879-883.

* The results for both diseases apply to the pediatric age group only.

HUMAN CHORIONIC GONADOTROPIN BETA SUBUNIT
(BETA-HCG URINE Hemagglutination)
1. Naryshkin S., Aw T.C., Filstein M., et al.: Comparison of the performance of serum and urine HCG immunoassays in the evaluation of gynecologic patients. *Ann. Emerg. Med.* 1985; 14(11):1074-1076.
2. Porres J.M., D'Ambra C., Lord D., et al.: Comparison of eight kits for the diagnosis of pregnancy. *Am. J. Clin. Path.* 1975; 64:452-463.

* N = 10 for sensitivity group.
* Consider possible variation between kits see paper #2.

HUMAN CHORIONIC GONADOTROPIN BETA SUBUNIT
(BETA-HCG SERUM - RIA)
1. Bryson, P.: B-Subunit of human chorionic gonadotropin, ultrasound, and ectopic pregnancy: A prospective study. *Am. J. Obstet. Gynecol.* 1985; 146(2):163-165.

2. Naryshkin S., Aw T.C., Filstein M., et al.: Comparison of the performance of serum and urine HCG immunoassays in the evaluation of gynecologic patients. *Ann. Emerg. Med.* 1985; 14(11):1074-1076.
3. Braunstein G.D., Vaitukaitis J.L., Carbone P.P., et al.: Ectopic production of human chorionic gonadotropin by neoplasms. *Ann. Int. Med.* 1973; 78(1):39-45.
4. Pecorelli S., Bianchi U.A., Cavagini A., et al.: CEA and beta-HCG as markers in gynecologic malignancies. *Cancer Treat. Rep.* 1979; 63:1183.
5. Klavins J.V.: Advances in biological markers for cancer. *Ann. Clin. Lab. Sci.* 1983;13(4):275-280.
6. Vaitukaitis J.L., Ross G.T., Braunstein G.D., et al.: Gonadotropins and their subunits: Basic and clinical studies. *Recent Progr. Hormone Res.* 1976; 32:289-331.

* 83 is the approximate specificity in the population suspected of having ectopic pregnancy (by history and clinical presentation). The test is very specific if intrauterine pregnancy can be ruled out.
* N = 26(combined from paper #1 and #2), N = 16 for seminoma, N = 18 for vulvar carcinoma.
* Type of tumor not specified in article.
* Population studied was Italian (except for ovarian cancer sensitivity N = 40).

HUMAN IMMUNODEFICIENCY VIRUS (HIV)

1. Carlson, J.R., Hinrichs, S.H., Levy, N.B., et al: Evaluation of commercial AIDS screening test kits. *Lancet,* 1985; 8442(1):1388.
2. Deinhardt, F., Eberle, J., Lutz, G.,: Sensitivity and specificity of eight commercial and one recombinant anti-HIV ELISA tests, *Lancet,* 1987; 8523(1):40.
3. Carlson, J.R., Bryant, M.L., Hinrichs, S.H., et al: AIDS serology testing in low- and high-risk groups, *JAMA,* 1985; 253(23):3405-3408.
4. Weiss, S. H., Goedert, J.J., Sarngadharan, M.G.: Screening test for T+HTLV-III (AIDS agent) antibodies, *JAMA,* 1985; 253(2):221-225.
5. Abramowicz, M., ed.: Screening for AIDS, *The Medical Letter,* 1985; 27: 29-30.
6. Sivak, S.L., Wormser, G.P.: Predictive value of a screening test for antibodies to HTLV-III, *Am. J. of Clin. Path.* 1986; 85(6):700-703.
7. Barnes, D.M.: New questions about AIDS test accuracy, *Science,* 1987; 238:884-885.

* Sensitivity of ELISA is high in patients with full AIDS syndrome. May
be as low as 33 in Western Blot positive blood donors.
* N = 15 for sensitivity of 80. There is much variation in sensitivity
between different commercial laboratories.

17-HYDROXYCORTICOSTEROIDS   (24 HOUR URINE)
1. Crapo L.: Cushings syndrome: A review of diagnostic tests,
   Metabol. 1979; 28(9):955-977.
2. Dunlap N.E., Grizzle W.E., Siegel A.L.: Cushing's syndrome, *Arch.
   Pathol. Lab. Med.* 1985; 109:222-229.

* Specificity is reported as 99 for "normal" controls and 73 for "obese
controls".

5-HYDROXYINDOLACETIC ACID, (5-HIAA) (24 HOUR URINE)
1.Feldman J.M.: Urinary serotonin in the diagnosis of carcinoid tumors.
   Clin. Chem. 1986; 32(5):840-844.

17-HYDROXYPROGESTERONE (RIA)
1. Wallace A.M., Beastall G.H., Cook B.J.: Neonatal screening for
   congenital adrenal hyperplasia: A program based on a novel direct
   radioimmunoassay for 17-hydroxyprogesterone in blood spots.
   Endocrin. 1985;108:299-308.
2. Cacciari B.A., Cassio A., Piazzi S., et al.: Neonatal screening for
   congenital adrenal hyperplasia. *Arch. of Dis. in Child.*,1983;
   58:803-806.

* N = 20 (21 Hydroxylase Deficiency is the most common cause of
congenital adrenal hyperplasia)
Reference #1 was done in Scotland, and #2 in Romania.

INSULIN ANTIBODIES (ELISA)
1. Telford M.E., Wisdom G.B.: Enzyme-immunoassay of anti-(bovine
   insulin) antibodies. *Biochem. Soc. Trans.*1979; 7:527-529.
2. Flynn S.D., Keren D.F., Torretti B., et al.: Factors affecting enzyme-
   linked immunosorbent assay (ELISA) for insulin antibodies in
   serum. *Clin. Chem.* 1981; 27(10):1753-1757.

* N = 19 in the control group for specificity.

IRON
1. Bassett M.L., Halliday J.W., Ferris R.A., et al.: Diagnosis of hemo-chromatosis in young subjects: Predictive accuracy of biochemical screening tests, *Gastroenterology* 1984; 87:628-633.
2. Borwein S.T., Ghent C.N., Valberg L.S.: Diagnostic efficacy of screening tests for hereditary hemochromatosis. *Can. Med. Assoc. J.* 1984; 131:895-901.
3. Kalmin N.D., Robson E.B., Bettigole R.E.: Serum ferritin and marrow iron stores. *N.Y. State J. Med.* 1978; June:1052-1055
4. Bainton D.F., Finch C.A.: The diagnosis of iron deficiency anemia. *Am J. Med.* 1964; 37:62-70.

* The sensitivity and specificity values for iron deficiency anemia were obtained from children ages 1-6 (ref. #1). There is further evidence of similar utility in adults (see ref.#3-4).

ISOAMYLASE
1. Steinberg, W.M., Goldstein, S.S., Davis, N.D., et. al.: Diagnostic assays in acute pancreatitis, a study of sensitivity and specificity. *Annals of Int. Med.* 1985; 102:576-580.

* The specificity of 85 is from a control group with abdominal pain.

JO, Nuclear Protein Antigens
1. Harmon, C.E.: Antinuclear antibodies in autoimmune disease, significance and pathogenicity, *Symposium on Clinical Immunology I,* 1985; 69(3):547-563.
2. Tan, E.M., Robinson, C.A., Nakamura, R.M.: ANAs in systemic rheumatic disease. *Postgrad. Med.* 1985; 78(3):141-148.
3. Tan, E.M.: *Advances in Immunology,* Kunkle and Dixon (eds.), Vol. 33, 1982; 172-185.
4. Nakamura, R.M., Rippey, J.H.: Quality assurance and proficiency testing for autoantibodies to nuclear antigen. *Arch. Pathol. Lab. Med.* 1985; 109:109-114.
5. Tan, E.M.: Antinuclear antibodies in diagnosis and management. *Hosp Pract.* 1983; 79-84.

KETOSTEROIDS,17, URINE
1. Dunlap N.E., Grizzle W.E., Siegel A.L.: Cushing's syndrome. *Arch. Pathol. Lab. Med.* 1985; 109:222-229.

LACTATE DEHYDROGENASE (SERIAL TESTS)

1. Lee, T.H., Goldman, L.: Serum enzyme assays in the diagnosis of acute myocardial infarction, *Annals of Int. Med,* 1986; 105:221-33.
2. Grande, P., Christiansen, C., Pedersen, A.: Optimal diagnosis in acute myocardial infarction, *Circulation,* 1980; 61(4)723-728.

* Serial tests defined as three samples obtained at 12 hour intervals.

LACTATE DEHYDROGENASE (SINGLE TEST)

1. Lee, T.H., Goldman, L.: Serum enzyme assays in the diagnosis of acute myocardial infarction, *Annals of Int. Med,* 1986; 105:221-33.
2. Lee, T.H., Weisberg, M.C., Cook, E.F., et al: Evaluation of creatine kinase and creatine kinase-MB for diagnosing myocardial infarction, *Arch Intern Med,* 1987; 147:115-121.

LDH ISOENZYMES

1. Vasudevan,G.,Mercer,D.W.,Varat, M.A.:Lactic dehydrogenase isoenzyme determination in the diagnosis of acute myocardial infarction. *Circulation* 1978; 57(6):1055-1057.
2. Wagner, G.S.,Roe,C.R.,Lee,L.E.:The Importance of Identification of the myocardial-specific isoenzyme of creatine phosphokinase (MB form) in the diagnosis of acute myocardial infarction. *Circulation.* 1973; XLVII:263-269.

LIPASE

1. Eckfeldt J.H., Kolars J.C., Elson M.K., et al.: Serum tests for pancreatitis in patients with abdominal pain. *Arch. Pathol. Lab. Med.* 1985; 109:316-319.
2. Steinberg W.M., Goldstein S.S., Davis N.D., et al.: Diagnostic assays in acute pancreatitis. *Ann. Int. Med.* 1985; 102:576-580.

* REFERENCE #1 showed lipase as 100% sensitive from the time of admission to the 2nd post admission day. Lipase was still positive in 50% 5-7 days post hospital admission (N = 9).
* The specificity was calculated from a group of patients with nonpancreatic acute abdominal pain.

LUTEINIZING HORMONE

1. Deutsch S., Krumholz B., Benjamin I.: The utility and selection of laboratory tests in the diagnosis of polycystic ovary syndrome. *J. Reprod. Med.* 1978; 20(5):275-282.
2. DeVane G.W., Czekala N.M., Judd H.L., *et al.*: Circulating gonadotropins, estrogens, and androgens in polycystic ovarian disease. *Am. J. Obstet. Gynecol.* 1975; 121(4):496-500.
3. Yen S.S., Tsai C.C., Vandenberg G.,et al.: Gonadotropin dynamics in patients with gonadal dysgenesis: A model for the study of gonadotropin regulation. *J. Clin. Endo. and Metab.* 1972; 35(6):897-904.

* Specificity was extrapolated from graphic data, the controls were composed of premenopausal females during days 1 and 2 of their menstrual cycle. In gonadal dysgenesis N =19.

MEAN CORPUSCULAR HEMOGLOBIN (MCH)

1. Hershko, C., Bar-Or, D., Gaziel, Y.: Diagnosis of iron deficiency anemia in a rural population of children. Relative usefulness of serum ferritin, red cell protoporphyrin, red cell indices, and transferrin saturation determinations. *Am J. of Clin. Nut.* 1981; 34:1600-1610.
2. Bainton D.F., Finch C.A.: The diagnosis of iron deficiency anemia. *Am J. Med.* 1964; 37:62-70.

* The sensitivity and specificity values for iron deficiency anemia were obtained from children ages 1-6 (ref. #1). There is further evidence of similar utility in adults (see ref.#2).

MEAN CORPUSCULAR VOLUME (MCV)

1. Hershko, C., Bar-Or, D., Gaziel, Y.: Diagnosis of iron deficiency anemia in a rural population of children. Relative usefulness of serum ferritin, red cell protoporphyrin, red cell indices, and transferrin saturation determinations. *Am. J. of Clin. Nut.* 1981; 34:1600-1610.
2. Bainton D.F., Finch C.A.: The diagnosis of iron deficiency anemia. *Am J. Med.* 1964; 37:62-70.

* The sensitivity and specificity values for iron deficiency anemia were obtained from children ages 1-6 (ref. #1). There is further evidence of similar utility in adults (see ref.#2).

METANEPHRINES (URINE)

1. Sjoerdsma A., Engleman K., Waldmann T.A.,et al.: Pheochromocytoma: Current concepts of diagnosis and treatment. *Ann. Int. Med.* 1966; 65:1302-26.
2. van Heerden J.A., Sheps S.G., Hamberger B., et al.: Pheochromocytoma: Current status and changing trends. *Surgery*, Apr. 1982; 91(4):367-73.
3. Bravo E.L., Tarazi R.C., Gifford R.W., et al.: Circulating and urinary catecholamines in pheochromocytoma: Diagnostic and pathophysiologic implications. *N.E.J.M.*, 1979; 301(13):682-686.

* Specificity estimated from values given from studies of normal controls. Reference #3 demonstrated a decrease in the specificity when the control group consisted of patients who had some signs of pheochromocytoma but were without laboratory evidence of disease.

5'-NUCLEOTIDASE

1. Ellis G., Goldberg D.M., Spooner R.J., et al Serum enzyme tests in diseases of the liver and biliary tree. *Am. J. Clin. Pathol.* 1978; 70(2):248-258.
2. Jonsson P., Bengtsson G., Carlsson G., et al.: Value of serum-5-nucleotidase, alkaline phosphatase and gamma-glutamyl transferase for prediction of hepatic metastases preoperatively in colorectal cancer. *Acta. Chir. Scand.* 1984; 150:419-423.
3. Kowlessar O.D., Haeffner L.J., Riley E.M., et al.: Comparative study of serum leucine aminopeptidase, 5-nucleotidase and non-specific alkaline phosphatase in diseases affecting the pancreas, hepatobiliary tree and bone. *Am. J. Med.* 1961; 31:231-237.
4. Batskis J.G.: The enzymes of the hepatobiliary tract: A biochemical and clinical comparison. *Ann. Clin. Lab. Sci.* 1974; 4(4):255-266.

* N = 20 for Carcinoma of the bile duct,N = 27 for intrahepatic cholestasis and N = 24 for primary biliary cirrhosis.
* N = 25 for sensitivity. Specificity group was not from a "normal population" but made up of patients with a previous diagnosis of colorectal cancer. 5-Nucleotidase was shown to be of very low sensitivity when < 1/4 of the liver volume is engaged by tumor and highly sensitive when > 3/4 of the liver volume is engaged by tumor. Population studied was Swedish.

PARATHYROID HORMONE (RIA) C - TERMINAL ASSAY,
N - TERMINAL ASSAY INTACT

1. Lufkin E.G., Kao P.C., Heath H.: Parathyroid hormone radioimmunoassays in the differential diagnosis of hypercalcemia due to primary
   hyperparathyroidism or malignancy. *Ann. Int. Med.* 1987;
   106(4):559-560.
2. Martin K. J., Hrusha K., Freitag J., et al.: Clinical utility of radioimmunoassays for parathyroid hormone. *Mineral Electrolyte
   Metab.* 1980; 3:283-290.
3. Lindall A.W., Elting J., Ells J., et al.: Estimation of biologically active
   intact parathyroid hormone in normal and hyperparathyroid sera by
   sequential N-terminal immunoextraction and midregion radioimmunoassay. *J Clin Endo & Metab.* 1983; 57(5):1007-1014.
4. Slatopolsky E., Martin K., Morrissey J. *et al.*: Current concepts of
   the metabolism and radioimmunoassay of parathyroid hormone.
   J. Lab. Clin. Med. 1982; 99(3):309-316.
5. Hawker C.D.: Parathyroid hormone: Radioimmunoassay and
   clinical interpretation. *Ann. Clin. Lab. Sci.* 1975; 5:383-397.
6. Arnaud C.D., Goldsmith R.S., Bordier P.J., et al.: Influence of
   immunoheterogeneity of circulating parathyroid hormone on
   results of radioimmunoassays of serum in man. *Amer. J. Med.*
   1974; 56:785-793.
7. Valsamis, J., Van Peborgh, J., Brauman, H.: Relative contribution
   of various expressions of cAMP excretion to other indices of
   parathyroid function, as tested by discriminant multivariate linear
   regression analysis. *Clin. Chem.* 1986; 32(7):1279-1284.

* Significant variation found due to differences between respective
laboratories and method of analysis. Variation may even be greater
depending on the studies included. Many reports show elevated
serum calcium in the evaluation of a patient with an elevated PTH.
N > or = 14 for above studies.

PARTIAL THROMBOPLASTIN TIME (PTT)

1. Nye S.W., Graham J.B., Brinkhous K.M.: The partial thromboplastin
   time as a screening test for the detection of latent bleeders. *Am.J.
   Med. Sci.* 1962; 243:279-87.
2. Suchman A.L., Griner P. F.: Diagnostic uses of the partial thromboplastin time and prothrombin time. *Ann. Int. Med.*1986; 104:810-816.
3. Lian C., Deykin D.: Diagnosis of von Willebrand's Disease. *Am. J of
   Med.* 1976; 60:344-356.

4. Hathaway W.E., Assmus S.L., Montgomery R.R.: Activated partial thromboplastin time and minor coagulopathies. *Am. Soc. Clin, Path.* 1979; 71(1):22-25.
5. Proctor R.R., Rapaport S.I.: The partial thromboplastin time with kaolin. *Am. J. Clin. Path.* 1961; 36(3):212-219.
6. Poller L.: Severe bleeding disorders in children with normal coagulation screening tests (letter). *Br. Med. J.* 1982; 285:377.

* Severe = 0-5% of normal, Moderate = 6-15%, Mild = 16-30%
* N = 11 for study yielding sensitivity of 100 and N = 33 for study yielding sensitivity of 48.
* N = 7 for Factor XII deficiency (from 2 papers), N = 1 for Factor XI deficiency and N = 3 for Factor XII deficiency.
* Specificity is calculated from a group of patients who were evaluated for abnormal bleeding, but did not have laboratory evidence of a bleeding disorder (reference #1) When plasma coagulant deficiencies (202 patients) are excluded from the 618 patients evaluated for bleeding, approximately 11% of the remaining patients demonstrate a prolonged PTT. These patients were accounted for by various other bleeding disorders.

PM-1, Nuclear Antigens

1. Harmon, C.E.: Antinuclear antibodies in autoimmune disease, significance and pathogenicity, *Symposium on Clinical Immunology I,* 1985; 69(3):547-563.
2. Tan, E.M., Robinson, C.A., Nakamura, R.M.: ANAs in systemic rheumatic disease. *Postgrad. Med.* 1985; 78(3):141-148.
3. Tan, E.M.: *Advances in Immunology,* Kunkle and Dixon (eds.), Vol. 33, 1982; 172-185.
4. Nakamura, R.M., Rippey, J.H.: Quality assurance and proficiency testing for autoantibodies to nuclear antigen. *Arch. Pathol. Lab. Med.* 1985; 109:109-114.
5. Tan, E.M.: Antinuclear antibodies in diagnosis and management. *Hosp Pract.* 1983; 79-84.

PORPHOBILINOGEN (Watson-Schwartz and Hoesch Methods)

1. Lamon J., With T.K., Redeker A.G.: The Hoesch test: Bedside screening in patients with suspected porphyria. *Clin. Chem.* 1974; 20(11):1438-1440.

* In porphyria, N = 7 in the calculation of sensitivity, for both tests. N = 19 for the specificity in both tests. The sensitivity was calculated to be 100 but false negatives have been reported.

POTASSIUM

1. Bravo, E.L., Tarazi, R.C., Dustan, H.P. et. al.: The changing clinical spectrum of primary aldosteronism. *Am. J. of Med.* 1983; 74:641-651.
2. Goldenberg, K., Snyder, D.K.: Screening for primary aldosteronism: hypokalemia in hypertensive patients. *J. of Gen. Int. Med.* 1986; 1:368-372.

* Sensitivity and specificity reported are for a potassium level of 3.5 used as a cutoff. Reference #2 suggests that using a cutoff value of 3.2 is optimal in mass screening for primary aldosteronism, due to adenoma (sensitivity = 90, specificity = 99).

PROTHROMBIN TIME (PT)

1. Marder V.J., Shulman N.R.: Clinical aspects of congenital factor VII deficiency. *Am. J. Med.* 1964; 37:182-194.
2. Owen C.A., Amundsen M.A., Thompson J.H.: Congenital deficiency of factor VII (hypoconvertinemia): Critical review of literature and report of three cases, with extensive pedigree study and effect of transfusions. *Am. J. Med.* 1964; 37:71-91.
3. Nye S.W., Graham J.B., Brinkhous K.M.: The partial thromboplastin time as a screening test for the detection of latent bleeders. *Am.J. Med. Sci.* 1962; 243:279-87.

* Prolonged prothrombin time has been demonstrated in other Factor deficiencies especially Factors V, X, and XII.

RANA (Immunodiffusion or Immunofluorescence)

1. Tan, E.M.: Antinuclear antibodies in diagnosis and management. *Hosp. Pract.* 1983; 79-84.
2. Nakamura R.M., Rippey J.H.: Quality assurance and proficiency testing for autoantibodies to nuclear antigen. *Arch. Pathol. Lab. Med.* 1985; 109:109-114.

RENIN (SUPPRESSED)

1. Bravo E.L., Tarazi R.C., Dustan H.P., et al.: The changing clinical spectrum of primary aldosteronism. *Am. J. Med,* 1983; 74:641-651.

* Suppressed = low Na intake for 4 days.
* Sensitivity and specificity are in relation to patients with essential
   hypertension and not to the general population where sensitivity
   would be lower and specificity would be higher.

Scl-70

1. Harmon C.E.: Antinuclear antibodies in autoimmune disease.
   Med. Clin. N. Am. 1985; 69(3):547-563.
2. Tan E.M., Robinson C.A., Nakamura R.M.: ANAs in systemic
   rheumatic disease: Diagnostic significance. *Postgrad. Med.* 1985;
   78(3):141-148.
3. Nakamura R.M., Rippey J.H.: Quality assurance and proficiency
   testing for autoantibodies to nuclear antigen, *Arch. Pathol. Lab.
   Med.* 1985; 109:109-114.
4. Powell D.L., Lipinski E., Steen V., et al.: Clinical associations of
   anti-Scl 70 antibody in patients with systemic sclerosis. *Arthritis
   Rheum.* 1984; 27:S19(#23).

SEROTONIN (URINE)

1. Feldman J.M.: Urinary Serotonin in the Diagnosis of Carcinoid
   Tumors. *Clin. Chem.* 1986; 32:840-844.
2. Engbaek F., Voldby B.: RIA of serotonin in cerebrospinal fluid,
   plasma, and serum. *Clin. Chem.* 1982; 624-628.
3. Taqari P.C., Boullin D.J., Davies C.I.: Simplified determination of
   serotonin in plasma by liquid chromatography with electrochemical
   detection. *Clin. Chem.* 1984; 30:131-135.

* In general patients with carcinoid tumors of the pancreas and
   bronchus show higher sensitivity (88) than carcinoid tumors in
   other locations, ie. midgut.

SS - A/Ro

1. Harmon C.E.: Antinuclear antibodies in autoimmune disease.
   Med. Clin. N. Am. 1985; 69(3):547-563.
2. Tan E.M., Robinson C.A., Nakamura R.M.: ANAs in systemic
   rheumatic disease: Diagnostic significance. *Postgrad. Med.*
   1985; 78(3):141-148.
3. Tan, E.M.: Antinuclear antibodies in diagnosis and management.
   Hosp Pract. 1983; 79-84.
4. Nakamura R.M., Rippey J.H.: Quality assurance and proficiency
   testing for autoantibodies to nuclear antigen, *Arch. Pathol. Lab.
   Med.* 1985; 109:109-114.

SS-B ANTIBODY

1. Harmon C.E.: Antinuclear antibodies in autoimmune disease. *Med. Clin. N. Am* 1985; 69(3):547-563.
2. Tan E.M., Robinson C.A., Nakamura R.M.: ANAs in systemic rheumatic disease: Diagnostic significance. *Postgrad. Med* 1985; 78(3):141-148.
3. Tan E.M.: Antinuclear antibodies in diagnosis and management. *Hosp. Pract.* Jan.1983.
4. Nakamura R.M., Rippey J.H.: Quality assurance and proficiency testing for autoantibodies to nuclear antigen. *Arch. Pathol. Lab. Med,* 1985; 109:109-114.

SS-DNA

1. Tan E.M.: Autoantibodies to nuclear antigens. *Advances in Immunology.* 1982; 33:172-175.
2. Stoller B.D., Levine L., Lohrer H.I., et al.: The antigenic determinants of denatured DNA reactive with systemic lupus erythematosus serum. *Proc. Natl. Acad. Sci. U.S.A.* 1962; 48:874-880.

THYROID ANTIMICROSOMAL ANTIBODIES (Hemagglutination)

1. Nobuyuki A., Hagen S.R., Yamada N., et al.: Measurement of circulating thyroid microsomal antibodies by the tanned red cell hemagglutination technique: Its usefulness in the diagnosis of autoimmune thyroid diseases. *Clin. Endo.* 1976; 5:115-125.
2. Abreau C.M., Vagenakis A. G., Roti E., et al., Clinical evaluation of a hemagglutination method for microsomal and thyroglobulin antibodies in autoimmune thyroid disease. *Ann. Cli. Lab Sci.* 1977; 7(1):73-78.

* N = 25 for primary hypothyroidism and N = 22 for nontoxic goiter.

THYROID ANTITHYROGLOBULIN ANTIBODIES (RIA)

1. Pinchera A., Mariotti S., Vitti P., et al.: Interference of serum thyro-globulin in the radioassay for serum antithyroglobulin antibodies. *J. Clin. Endocr. and Metab.* 1977; 45:1077-1088.
2. Mori T., Kriss J.P.: Measurements by competitive binding radioassay or serum antimicrosomal and anti-thyroglobulin antibodies in Graves' disease and other thyroid disorders. *J. Clin. Endocr. and Metab,* 1971; 33:688-698.

3. Levy W., Gupta M.K., Valenzuela R., et al.: A simple semiquanti-
tative radiometric measurement of antithyroglobulin antibodies in
human serum. *Clin. Physiol. Biochem.* 1984; 2:198-204.
4. Ericsson U., Christensen S.B., Thorell J.I.: A high prevalence of
thyroglobulin autoantibodies in adults with and without thyroid
disease as measured with a sensitive solid-phase immunosorbent
radioassay. *Clin. Immuno. and Immunopath.* 1985; 37:154-162.

* The results reported are from reference #1 (population studied was
Italian). The other references lend support to the reported data when
the cut offs are similar levels.
* N = 18 for Hashimoto's thyroiditis, N = 13 for idiopathic myxedema and
N = 9 for pituitary hypothyroidism.
* Reference #4 demonstrates possible differences in sensitivity and
specificity between sexes. This is not as apparent when the cut
off is increased to the level used in reference #1.

THYROID - ANTITHYROGLOBULIN ANTIBODIES
(HEMAGGLUTINATION)

1. Pinchera A., Mariotti S., Vitti P., et al.: Interference of serum thyroglobulin in the radioassay for serum antithyroglobulin antibodies.
J. Clin. Endocrinol. Metab. 1977; 45:1077-1088.
2. Ericsson U., Christensen S.B.: Thorell J.I.: A high prevalence of
thyroglobulin autoantibodies in adults with and without thyroid
disease as measured with a sensitive solid-phase immunosorbent radioassay. *Clin. Immuno. and Immunopath.* 1985;
37:154-162.

* The results reported are from reference #1 (population studied was
Italian).
* N = 18 for Hashimoto's thyroiditis, N = 13 for idiopathic myxedema
and N = 9 for pituitary hypothyroidism.
* Reference #2 demonstrates possible differences in sensitivity and
specificity between sexes.

THYROID RELATED HORMONE TESTS (TSH-RIA,
TSH-IRMA, TOTAL T4, FREE T4, FREE T4 UPTAKE, TOTAL
T3, FREE T3, FREE T3 INDEX)

1. Ericsson U.B., Fernlund P., Thorell J.I.: Evaluation of the usefulness
of a sensitive immunoradiometric assay for thyroid stimulation
hormone as a first-line thyroid function test in an unselected patient
population. *Scand. J. Clin. lab. Invest.* 1987; 47:215-221.

2. Goldstein B.J., Mushlin A.I.: Use of a single thyroxine test to evaluate ambulatory medical patients for suspected hypothyroidism. *J. Gen. Int. Med.* 1987; 2:20-24.
3. Caldwell G., Gow S.M., Sweeting V.M., et al.: A new strategy for thyroid function testing. *The Lancet.* 1985; May 18:1117-1119.
4. Wilke T.J., Eastment H.T.: Discriminative ability of tests for free and total thyroid hormones in diagnosing thyroid disease. *Clin. Chem.* 1986; 32(9):1746-1750.
5. Allen K.R., Watson D.: Thyrotropin as the initial screening test for thyroid function. *Clin. Chem.* 1984; 30(3):502-503.
6. Penny M.D., O'Sullivan D.J.: Total or free thyroxin as a primary test of thyroid function. *Clin. Chem.* 1987; 33(1):170-171.
7. Tunbridge W.M.G., Evered D.C., Hall R., et al.: The spectrum of thyroid disease in a community: The Whickham survey. *Clin. Endo.* 1977; 7:481-493.

* The TSH-RIA test for hypothyroidism has been shown to be less specific for females (93) than for males (97). See Ref.#7.
* The specificities for TSH-IRMA, Total T4, Free T4 Index, and total T3 have been determined using documented euthyroid controls (the higher specificity) and for controls made up of a mixture of documented euthyroid patients and patients with other thyroid diseases (the lower specificity). The latter control mixture may be similar to that found at a tertiary care hospital. See Ref.#1.

TOTAL IRON BINDING CAPACITY (TIBC)

1. Hershko, C., Bar-Or, D., Gaziel, Y.: Diagnosis of iron deficiency anemia in a rural population of children. Relative usefulness of serum ferritin, red cell protoporphyrin, red cell indices, and transferrin saturation determinations. *Am J. of Clin. Nut.* 1981; 34:1600-1610.
2. Walsh J.R., Fredreckson M.: Serum ferritin, free erythrocyte protoporphyrin, and urinary iron excretion in patients with iron disorders. *Am. J. Med. Sci.* 1977; 273(3):293-300.
3. Kalmin N.D., Robson E.B., Bettigole R.E.: Serum ferritin and marrow iron stores. *N.Y. State J. Med.* 1978; June:1052-1055.

* The sensitivity and specificity values for iron deficiency anemia were obtained from children ages 1-6 (ref. #1). There is further evidence of similar utility in adults (see refs. 2+3).

TOXICOLOGY, URINE

1. Hansen H.J., Caudill S.P., Boone J.: Crisis in drug testing: Results of CDC blind study. *J.A.M.A*, 1985; 243(16):2382-2387.

* The wide range in values represents differences in performance between the laboratories used (reference #1).

TRANSFERRIN SATURATION

1. Bassett M.L., Halliday J.W., Ferris R.A., et al.: Diagnosis of hemo-chromatosis in young subjects: Predictive accuracy of biochemical screening tests, *Gastroenterology* 1984; 87:628-633.
2. Borwein S.T., Ghent C.N., Valberg L.S.: Diagnostic efficacy of screening tests for hereditary hemochromatosis. *Can. Med. Assoc. J.* 1984; 131:895-901.
3. Griner P.F., Mayewski R.J., Mushlin A.I., et al.: Selection and interpretation of diagnostic tests and procedures principles and applications. *Ann. Int. Med.* 1981; 94(part 2):553-599.
4. Hershko C., Bar-Or D., Gaziel Y., et al.: Diagnosis of iron deficiency anemia in a rural population of children. Relative usefulness of serum ferritin, red cell protoporphyrin, red cell indices and transferrin saturation determinations. *Am. J. Clin Nutrition.* 1981; 34:1600-1610.
5. Bainton D.F., Finch C.A.: The diagnosis of iron deficiency anemia. *Am. J. Med.* 1964; 37:62-70.
6. Hershko, C., Bar-Or, D., Gaziel, Y.: Diagnosis of iron deficiency anemia in a rural population of children. Relative usefulness of serum ferritin, red cell protoporphyrin, red cell indices, and transferrin saturation determinations. *Am. J. of Clin. Nut.* 1981; 34:1600-1610.
7. Walsh J.R., Fredreckson M.: Serum ferritin, free erythrocyte proto-porphyrin, and urinary iron excretion in patients with iron disorders. *Am. J. Med. Sci.* 1977; 273(3):293-300.
8. Mazza J., Barr R.M., McDonald J.W., et. al.: Usefulness of the serum ferritin concentration in the detection of iron deficiency in a general hospital. *CMA. J.* 1978; 119:884-886.
9. Kalmin N.D., Robson E.B., Bettigole R.E.: Serum ferritin and marrow iron stores. *N.Y. State J. Med.* 1978; June:1052-1055.

* The sensitivity and specificity values for iron deficiency anemia were obtained from children ages 1-6 (ref. #6). There is further evidence of similar utility in adults (see refs. 6-9). The specificity of ferritin is

thought to be higher in adults vs.transferrin (96 vs. 63 respectively, see ref. #8).
* The sensitivity value provided is from "young" patients (<35yrs old). The specificity was derived from first degree relatives of hemochromatosis probands who were not homozygous but ≥16% were heterozygous.
* Differences in sensitivity and specificity have been shown using different cut off values (see reference #2, no discrimination for age noted).

TRYPSINOGEN

1. Steinberg, W.M., Goldstein, S.S., Davis, N.D., et. al.: Diagnostic assays in acute pancreatitis, a study of sensitivity and specificity. *Annals of Int. Med*. 1985; 102:576-580.

* The specificity of 82 is from a control group of patients with abdominal pain.

VASOACTIVE INTESTINAL PEPTIDE

1. Bloom S.R., Vasoactive intestinal peptide, the major mediator of the WDHA (pancreatic cholera) syndrome: Value of measurement in diagnosis and treatment. *Dig. Dis*. 1978; 23(4):373-376.
2. Bloom S.R., Polak J.M., Pearse A.G., et al.:Vasoactive intestinal peptide and watery-diarrhea syndrome. *Lancet* 1973; 2:14-16.
3. Mitchell S.J., Bloom S.R.: Measurement of fasting and postprandial plasma VIP in man. *Gut* 1978; 19:1043-1048.
4. Long R.G., Bryant M.G., Mitchell S.J., et al.: Clinicopathological study of pancreatic and ganglioneuroblastoma tumours secreting vasoactive intestinal polypeptide (vipomas), *Br. Med. J.* 1981; 282:1767-1771.

* N = 10 for ganglioneuroblastoma.

VDRL

1. Moyer, N.P., Hudson., J.D., Hausler, W.J.: Evaluation of the hemagglutination treponemal test for syphilis. *J. of Clin. Microbio.* 1984; 19(6):849-852.
2. Moyer, N.P., Hudson., J.D., Hausler, W.J.: Evaluation of the bio-enzabead test for syphilis. *J. of Clin. Microbio.* 1987; 25(4):619-623.
3. Deacon, W.E., Lucas, J.B., Price, E.V.: Fluorescent treponemal antibody-absorption (FTA-ABS) test for syphilis. *J.A.M.A.* 1966; 198(6):156-160.

4. Hart, G.: Syphilis tests in diagnostic and therapeutic decision making. *Ann. of Int. Med.* 1986; 104:368-376.

* N = 24 for early-latent syphilis.
* Specificity of 84 is calculated from control group comprised of "sick patients" (reference #4).

VMA (URINE)

1. Kaufman B.H., Telander R.L., van Heerden J.A.: Pheochromocytoma in the pediatric age group: Current status. *J. Ped. Surg.* 1983; 18(6):879-883.
2. Sjoerdsma A., Engelman K., Waldmann T.A., et al.: Pheochromocytoma: Current concepts of diagnosis and treatment. *Ann. Int. Med,* 1966; 65(6):1302-1326.
3. van Heerden J.A., Sheps S.G., Hamberger B., *et al.*: Pheochromocytoma: Current status and changing trends. *Surgery* 1982; 91(4):367-73.
4. Bravo E.L., Tarazi R.C., Gifford R.W., et al.: Circulating and urinary catecholamines in pheochromocytoma: Diagnostic and pathophysiologic implications. *N. E.J. M.* 1979; 301(13):682-686.
5. Tuchman M., Ramnaraine M.L., Woods W.G., et al.: Three years of experience with random urinary homovanillic and vanillylmandelic acid levels in the diagnosis of neuroblastoma. *Peds.* 1987; 79(2):203-205.
6. Woods W.G., Tuchman M.: Neuroblastoma: The case for screening infants in North America. *Peds.* 1987; 79(6):869-873.
7. Johnsonbaugh R.E., Cahill R.: Screening procedures for neruoblastoma: False-negative results. *Peds.* 1975; 56(2):267-270.
8. Matsumoto M., Anazawa A., Suzuki K., et al.: Urine mass screening for neuroblastoma by high performance liquid chromatography (HPLC). *Pediatr. Res.* 1985; 19:625.
9. Piasano J.J., Crout J.R., Abraham D.: Determination of 3-methoxy-4-hydroxymandelic acid in urine. *Clin. Chima. ACTA,* 1962; 7:285-291.

* The method of analysis reference#1 has sensitivity of 95 which is for specific extraction and periodate oxidation (described in ref #8) with some modifications.
* Sensitivity is from reference#1.Capillary gas chromatography was the method of analysis. The sensitivity may be much lower with other methods of testing (*ie* spot test ref. #2 and #3).

* Specificity varies with test method. Reference #4 reports a decrease in the specificity when the control group consists of patients with some signs of pheochromocytoma but without laboratory evidence. (The method of analysis in reference #4 was the specific extraction and periodate oxidation described in reference #9.

SECTION V

Cost Analysis of Selected Tests

H. Verdain Barnes, M.D.

LABORATORY TEST	EAST	SOUTH/MIDWEST	NORTH/CENTRAL	WEST	AVERAGE Cost/Test	RANGE
ACID PHOSPHATASE	$11.00	$11.25	$12.25	$18.25	$13.19	$11.00 - $18.25
ALANINE AMINOTRANSFERASE	$6.50	$6.50	$5.90	$6.13	$6.26	$5.90 - $6.50
ALDOSTERONE NONSUPPRESSIBLE (Serum)	$69.75	$84.25	$95.00	$89.67	$84.67	$69.75 - $95.00
ALDOSTERONE NONSUPPRESSIBLE (Urine)	$69.75	$84.25	98.00	$100.67	$84.89	$69.75 - $100.67
ALKALINE PHOSPHATASE	$6.75	$6.75	$5.90	$7.75	$6.79	$5.90 - $7.75
ALPHA-FETOPROTEIN	$33.00	$43.50	$40.00	$43.67	$40.04	$33.00 - $43.67
AMMONIA	$25.25	$33.50	$32.00	$35.65	$31.60	$25.25 - $35.65
AMYLASE	$8.75	$10.75	$8.80	$11.42	$9.93	$8.75 - $11.42
ANTI DNA, Double Stranded	$30.50	$30.25	$32.00	$34.92	$31.92	$30.25 - $34.92
ANTI DNA, Single Stranded	$21.50	$30.25	$32.00	$42.17	$31.48	$21.50 - $42.17
ANTI-Histone Antibody	$45.75	$37.00	$40.00	$59.00	$45.44	$37.00 - $59.00
ANTI-NUCLEAR ANTIBODY	$19.25	$25.50	$19.95	$29.48	$23.55	$19.25 - $29.48
ANTI-RIBONUCLEAR PROTEIN	$44.00	$46.00	$44.00	$55.33	$47.33	$44.00 - $55.33
ANTI-SM ANTIBODY	$44.00	$28.00	$44.00	$37.42	$38.36	$28.00 - $44.00
ANTITHROMBIN III	$20.50	$32.50	-	$54.33	$35.78	$20.50 - $54.33
ASPARTATE AMINOTRANSFERASE	$6.25	$6.50	$5.90	$7.33	$6.50	$5.90 - $7.33
B-12	$27.25	$32.25	$25.20	$37.50	$30.55	$25.20 - $37.50
BILE ACIDS	$24.25	$27.50	-	$34.00	$28.58	$24.25 - $34.00
BILIRUBIN, TOTAL	$10.00	$6.50	$5.90	$7.67	$7.52	$5.90 - $10.00
CALCIUM	$6.00	$6.50	$5.90	$7.33	$6.43	$5.90 - $7.33
cAMP, URINE	$48.50	$56.00	$56.00	$84.67	$61.29	$48.50 - $84.67
CAROTENE	$18.75	$17.75	$23.75	$28.65	$22.23	$17.75 - $28.65
CATECHOLAMINES	$73.75	$97.75	$89.50	$74.33	$83.83	$73.75 - $97.75
CENTROMERE/KINETOCHORE	$31.25	$32.00	$32.00	$38.00	$33.31	$31.25 - $38.00
CERULOPLASMIN	$18.00	$18.25	$25.00	$24.65	$21.48	$18.00 - $25.00
COPPER	$17.75	$26.00	$37.50	$31.17	$28.11	$17.75 - $37.50
COPPER, URINE	$21.00	$24.50	$37.50	$32.00	$28.75	$21.00 - $37.50
CORTISOL, 24 hour FREE URINE	$36.00	$41.00	$42.00	$49.42	$42.11	$36.00 - $49.42
CORTISOL, PLASMA	$24.25	$37.25	$29.95	$33.83	$31.32	$24.25 - $37.25
C PEPTIDE	$38.25	$37.75	$59.50	$49.00	$46.13	$37.75 - $59.50

LABORATORY TEST	EAST	SOUTH/ MIDWEST	NORTH/ CENTRAL	WEST	AVERAGE Cost/Test	RANGE
C REACTIVE PROTEIN	$7.25	$11.00	$7.90	$17.25	$10.85	$7.25 - $17.25
CREATINE PHOSPHOKINASE MB FRA	$36.75	$26.00	$28.00	$34.58	$31.33	$26.00 - $36.75
CREATINE PHOSPHOKINASE	$11.25	$11.00	$5.90	$12.47	$10.16	$5.90 - $12.47
DEXAMETHASONE SUPPRESSION TEST SINGLE DOSE	$25.50	$36.75	$29.00	$40.17	$32.86	$25.50 - $40.17
FECAL FAT-QUALATATIVE	$10.50	$11.25	$8.80	$18.25	$12.20	$8.80 - $18.25
FIBRINOGEN/FIBRIN	$15.00	$15.00	$19.65	$14.33	$16.00	$14.33 - $19.65
5 NUCLEOTIDASE	$24.50	$21.25	$26.00	$23.58	$23.83	$21.25 - $26.00
5-HIAA (Urine)	$18.50	$80.75	$42.50	$43.32	$46.27	$18.50 - $80.75
FOLIC ACID	$26.75	$32.50	$25.20	$28.58	$28.26	$25.20 - $32.50
FTA-ABS	$19.00	$21.00	$26.50	$31.32	$24.46	$19.00 - $31.32
GAMMA GLUTAMYL TRANSPEPTIDASE	$8.00	$9.25	$5.90	$11.08	$8.56	$5.90 - $11.08
GROWTH HORMONE, FASTING	$33.00	$35.00	$42.00	$40.13	$37.53	$33.00 - $42.00
HAPTOGLOBULIN	$24.00	$26.00	$28.90	$37.82	$29.18	$24.00 - $37.82
HEMOGLOBIN A1C	$18.50	$21.50	$14.90	$20.25	$18.79	$14.90 - $21.50
HEPATITIS A IgM ANTI-HAV	$23.75	$28.00	$18.00	$30.32	$25.02	$18.00 - $30.32
HEPATITIS A TOTAL Anti-HAV	$23.75	$24.25	$16.00	$29.58	$23.40	$16.00 - $29.58
HEPATITIS B Anti-HBc	$23.75	$24.25	$16.00	$29.67	$23.42	$16.00 - $29.67
HEPATITIS B Anti-HBe	$23.75	$24.25	$22.00	$26.00	$24.00	$22.00 - $26.00
HEPATITIS B Anti-HBs	$23.75	$24.25	$16.00	$21.25	$21.31	$16.00 - $24.25
HEPATITIS B HBeAg	$23.75	$24.25	$22.00	$23.25	$23.31	$22.00 - $24.25
HEPATITIS B HBs-Ag	$15.25	$20.50	$13.00	$21.25	$17.50	$13.00 - $21.25
ANTI EBV ANTIBODY	$15.00	$34.50	$8.75	$38.17	$24.11	$8.75 - $38.17
HLA-B27	$50.00	$52.00	$54.00	$49.33	$51.33	$49.33 - $54.00
HUMAN CHORIONIC GONADOTROPIN BETA SUBUNIT	$14.75	$17.25	$16.50	-	$16.17	$14.75 - $17.25
HUMAN IMMUNO DEFICIENCY VIRUS	$20.50	$31.25	$14.00	-	$21.92	$14.00 - $31.25
HVA 24 HOUR URINE	$55.75	$52.00	$72.15	$55.75	$58.91	$52.00 - $72.15
17 HYDROXYCORTICOSTEROIDS 24 HOUR URINE	$25.25	$33.00	$59.50	$42.42	$40.04	$25.25 - $59.50

LABORATORY TEST	EAST	SOUTH/MIDWEST	NORTH/CENTRAL	WEST	AVERAGE Cost/Test	RANGE
17 HYDROXYPROGESTERONE	$49.00	$48.50	$60.00	$56.69	$53.55	$48.50 - $60.00
INSULIN ANTIBODIES (ELISA)	$41.25	$50.75	$79.50	$63.33	$58.71	$41.25 - $79.50
17 KETOSTEROIDS 24 HOUR URINE	$26.25	$24.75	$39.50	$33.92	$31.11	$24.75 - $39.50
LDH ISOENZYMES	$25.50	$37.75	$32.00	$38.98	$33.56	$25.50 - $38.98
LACTATE DEHYDROGENASE	$6.25	$6.00	$5.90	$8.33	$6.62	$5.90 - $8.33
LIPASE	$9.00	$10.00	$15.75	$22.42	$14.29	$9.00 - $22.42
LUTEINIZING HORMONE	$33.00	$45.25	$36.40	$41.65	$39.08	$33.00 - $45.25
METANEPHRINES	$44.00	$34.50	$61.50	$46.42	$46.61	$34.50 - $61.50
MONOSPOT	$10.50	$9.00	$8.75	$9.75	$9.50	$8.75 - $10.50
PARATHYROID HORMONE	$102.75	$97.25	$99.75	$94.17	$98.48	$94.17 - $102.75
PARTIAL THROMBOPLASTIN TIME (aPTT)	$8.75	$10.75	$14.00	$12.00	$11.38	$8.75 - $14.00
PORPHOBILINOGEN	$16.75	$17.00	$39.50	$18.33	$22.90	$16.75 - $39.50
POTASSIUM	$5.50	$5.75	$4.75	$7.08	$5.77	$4.75 - $7.08
PROTHROMBIN TIME (PT)	$6.50	$6.75	$7.00	$8.00	$7.06	$6.50 - $8.00
RANA (RheumatoidArthritis associated Nuclear Antigens)	$32.00	$9.25	$10.80	$32.92	$21.24	$9.25 - $32.92
RENIN	$43.50	$48.50	$66.50	$49.82	$52.08	$43.50 - $66.50
SCL-70	$29.50	-	-	$51.25	$40.38	$29.50 - $51.25
SEROTONIN		$118.75	$117.50	$86.32	$107.52	$86.32 - $118.75
SS-A ANTIBODY	$40.75	$51.75	$41.00	$44.42	$44.48	$40.75 - $51.75
SS-B ANTIBODY	$40.75	$51.75	$41.00	$49.92	$45.86	$40.75 - $51.75
THYROID ANTIMICROSOMAL ANTIBODIES	$28.00	$18.50	$26.00	$31.65	$26.04	$18.50 - $31.65
THYROID ANTITHYROGLOBULIN ANTIBODIES (RIA)	$17.00	$18.50	$26.00	$33.48	$23.75	$17.00 - $33.48
TOXICOLOGY URINE	$68.25	$54.00	$30.00	$46.67	$49.73	$30.00 - $68.25
TRANSFERRIN	$23.00	$28.50	$26.00	$29.00	$26.63	$23.00 - $29.00
VANILLYMANDELIC ACID (VMA URINE)	$29.00	$31.75	$63.50	$46.92	$42.79	$29.00 - $63.50
VASOACTIVE INTESTINAL PEPTIDE		$78.00	$106.50	$96.50	$93.67	$78.00 - $106.50
VDRL	$5.50	$6.50	$6.00	$13.67	$7.92	$5.50 - $13.67
WESTERN BLOT	$52.50	$43.25	$75.50	$58.33	$57.40	$43.25 - $75.50

Index